To Chris with much love from
Terry
GW00691567

Aromatherapy
Secrets

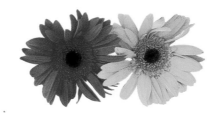

Aromatherapy Secrets

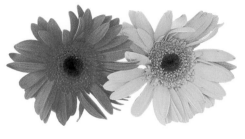

Nerys Purchon

Styling by Louise Owens
Photography by Quentin Bacon

Hodder & Stoughton

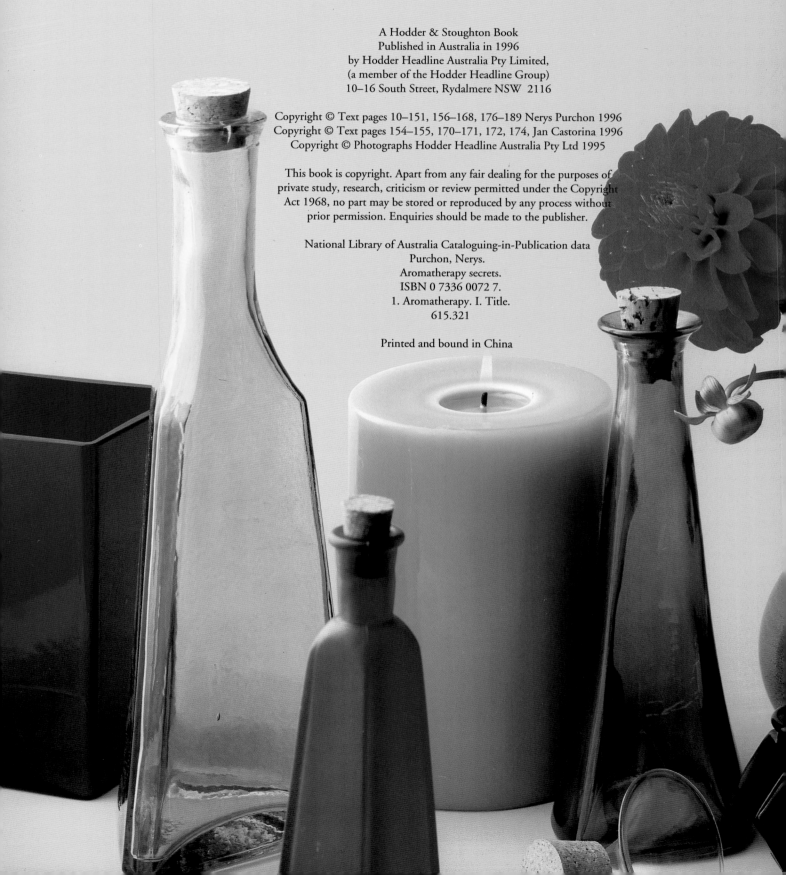

Editors: Pamela Allardice and Jan Castorina
Designer: Liz Seymour
Layout Artist: Raylee Sloane
Illustrations: Dhenu Jennifer Clary
Stylist's Assistants: Amanda Greenfield, Michael Wilkinson

A Hodder & Stoughton Book
Published in Australia in 1996
by Hodder Headline Australia Pty Limited,
(a member of the Hodder Headline Group)
10–16 South Street, Rydalmere NSW 2116

Copyright © Text pages 10–151, 156–168, 176–189 Nerys Purchon 1996
Copyright © Text pages 154–155, 170–171, 172, 174, Jan Castorina 1996
Copyright © Photographs Hodder Headline Australia Pty Ltd 1995

This book is copyright. Apart from any fair dealing for the purposes of
private study, research, criticism or review permitted under the Copyright
Act 1968, no part may be stored or reproduced by any process without
prior permission. Enquiries should be made to the publisher.

National Library of Australia Cataloguing-in-Publication data
Purchon, Nerys.
Aromatherapy secrets.
ISBN 0 7336 0072 7.
1. Aromatherapy. I. Title.
615.321

Printed and bound in China

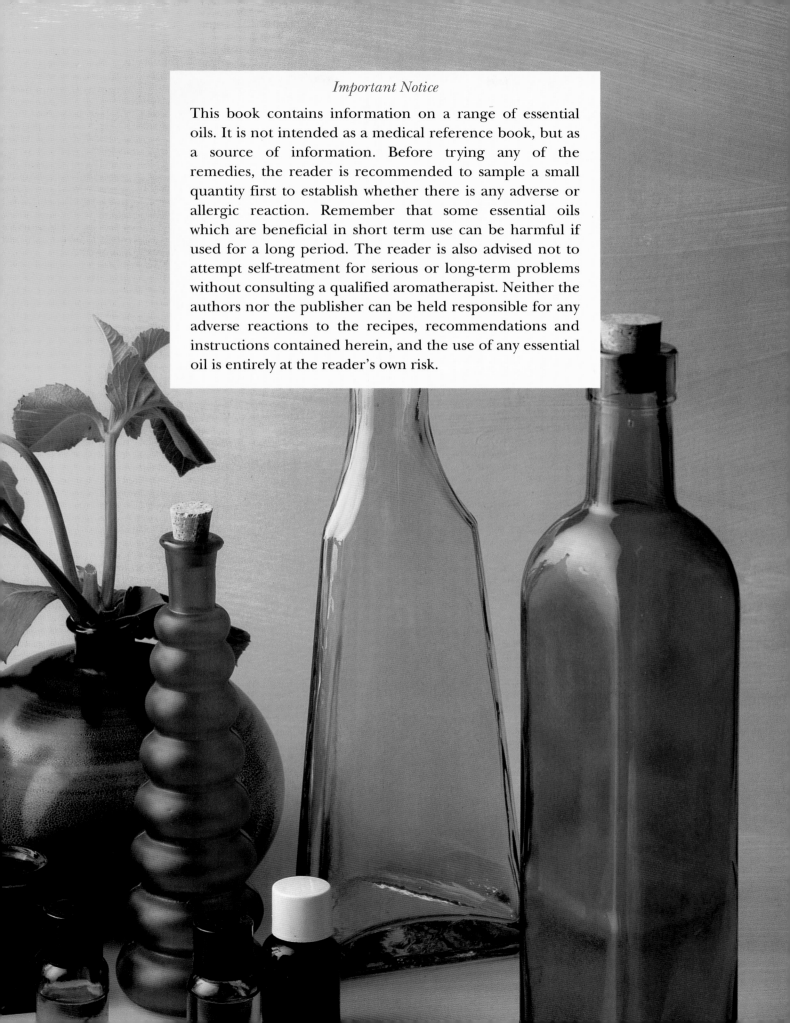

Important Notice

This book contains information on a range of essential oils. It is not intended as a medical reference book, but as a source of information. Before trying any of the remedies, the reader is recommended to sample a small quantity first to establish whether there is any adverse or allergic reaction. Remember that some essential oils which are beneficial in short term use can be harmful if used for a long period. The reader is also advised not to attempt self-treatment for serious or long-term problems without consulting a qualified aromatherapist. Neither the authors nor the publisher can be held responsible for any adverse reactions to the recipes, recommendations and instructions contained herein, and the use of any essential oil is entirely at the reader's own risk.

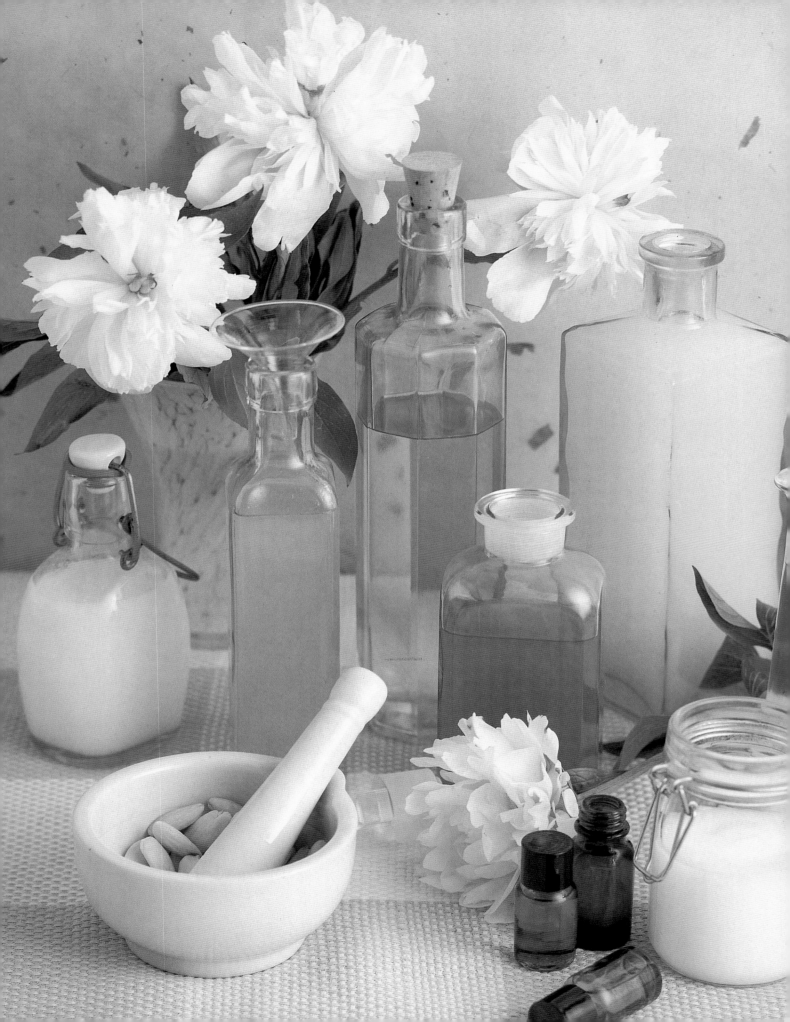

Contents

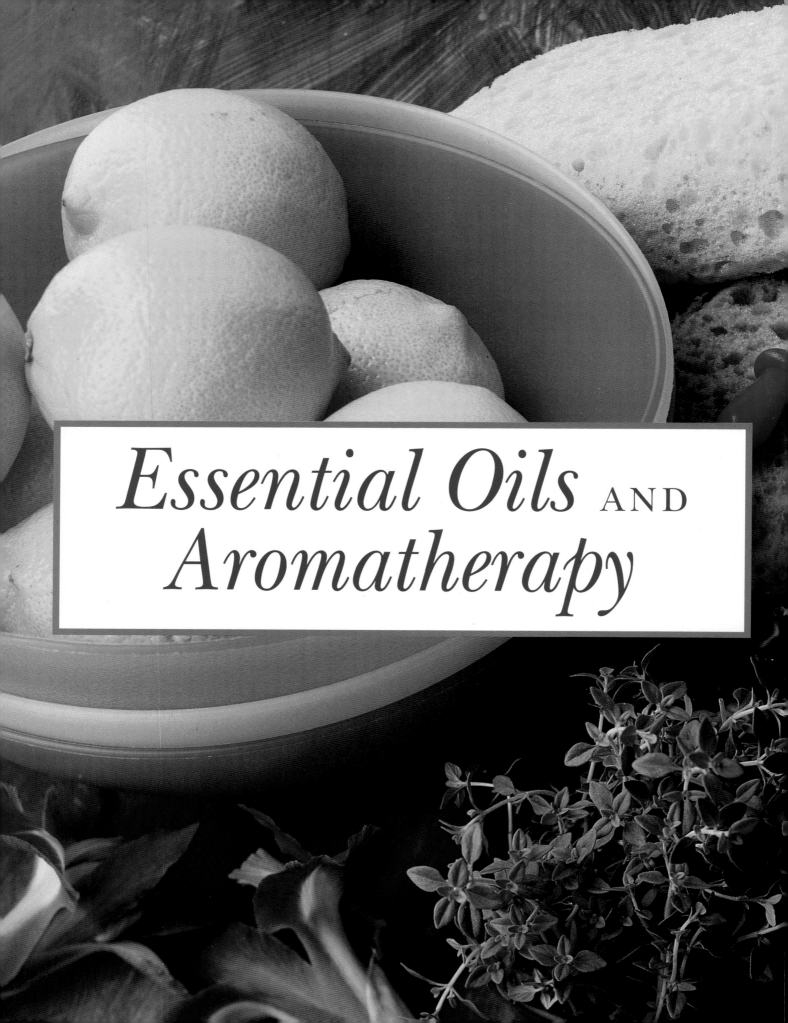

Essential Oils AND Aromatherapy

TIP

Essential oils have been described as the 'life force' or essence of plants. Buy only the purest, highest quality oils you can find.

Essential oils have been variously described as the 'life force' or 'essence' of plants. The most wonderful thing about essential oils is that they are available to everyone and, once you understand and observe the basic concepts, they are very simple to use. The essential oils differ from cooking or 'fixed' oils in that they are not oily to the touch, and they evaporate when exposed to air.

Aromatherapy is a method of employing the essential oils extracted from plants to protect, heal and beautify. The best known way to employ the oils is through massage but, as you will see in this book, there are many more ways to use the oils.

The use of essential oils for healing, deodorising or beautifying, and their use in religious ceremonies, has been recorded for centuries. However, the use of herbs, essential oils and other natural methods of healing fell into disfavour when scientists discovered ways of synthesising drugs. These days, essential oils are attracting more attention and are emerging as scientifically proven and accepted remedies: folklore and mystique are joining hands with modern scientific research.

We now understand how and why certain essential oils heal, but the actions of many still remain a mystery. Sceptics will scoff if you are unable to offer a 'scientific' explanation as to how the oils work, and yet the orthodox medical profession still cannot explain how aspirin, for instance, performs its pain-killing function!

The oils should not be used internally, unless prescribed by a qualified practitioner. It was Paracelsus (1493–1541) who said: "All is poison, nothing is poison". This is particularly true when applied to the use of essential oils. Oils taken over too long a period or in too great an amount can create or exacerbate the symptoms which they are supposed to treat. Peppermint oil, for instance, is useful for easing nausea and certain types of headache; however, if it is used excessively, it can then cause the headaches and nausea.

The cautions and suggestions for quantities to use which I have provided in this book need to be carefully observed. The difference in action between 1 and 2 drops is very great—1 drop of essential oil equals 1 cup (155ml/5fl oz) of herbal infusion!

This book is not intended to take the place of the advice of a health professional, and we need to remember that even simple symptoms can mask serious complaints. If symptoms are severe or of long duration, the condition needs to be assessed professionally. What the oils can do is to help us to treat everyday ailments: to strengthen our immune system, organs and glands, to fight bacteria, fungi and viruses, to lower our stress levels and to tone, relax and strengthen our muscles.

I would urge you to buy only the purest, highest quality oils you can find. With the upsurge in popularity of aromatherapy, there are many synthetic and adulterated oils appearing in the marketplace. Synthetic oils do not have the therapeutic value of the genuine ones and could, in fact, prove to be harmful. These oils are often labelled 'Fragrant Oil', 'Perfume Oil' or 'Compound Oil'. Instead, look for labels which say '100% Pure Essential Oil' or, in some cases where the oil is very expensive, you may find that the label reads '2.5% (or 3%) Essential Oil in a Carrier Oil'. This is usually the way in which very costly oils such as rose, chamomile and neroli are sold, and is perfectly acceptable.

When you venture out to buy your first oils they may appear expensive. However, when you consider how little is used and how much plant material is required to yield a tiny amount of oil (thyme, for instance, yields approximately only 200ml ($6\frac{1}{2}$fl oz) of essential oil from 1000kg (50lb) of plant material!) you will realise that you are getting value for money. After all, this purchase may be an investment in the future good health and well-being of both you and your family.

Guide to Measures

In some countries they use metric measures, in others imperial measures, and many like to use handy cup and spoon measures. In Australia, we use metric measures and cup and spoon measures approved by the Standards Association of Australia.

- The metric measuring cup holds 250ml
- The metric measuring tablespoon holds 20ml
- The metric measuring teaspoon holds 5ml

The conversions given in the recipes in this book are approximate. Any differences should not make any noticeable difference to these recipes.

- Measure accurately
- Label carefully
- Store properly
- Blend correct proportions
- Use dark glass bottles
- Be aware of cautions for specific oils

How to Store the Oils

- Keep the oils in dark-coloured bottles—blue or amber are good.
- Keep the bottles as full as possible, as air can cause spoilage.
- Label the bottles carefully as some oils smell very similar.
- Store the oils in a box in a dark, dry, cool place. Do not store them in a refrigerator, as this will thicken them and possibly introduce moisture.

Blending Guide

The essential oils must be measured very accurately as they are immensely powerful. If a recipe says to use 2 drops, then 4 drops will certainly not be better! Droppers or syringes and glass or plastic measures may be bought from pharmacies.

The following list is a general guide to amounts to use. Individual recipes may contain more or less essential oil.

Massage oils	2–2.5%
Massage creams	2–2.5%
Fomentations and compresses	10 drops to 100ml ($3\frac{1}{3}$fl oz) water
Ointments	3%
Lotions	1–$1\frac{1}{2}$%
Baths	10 drops maximum
Footbaths	4–6 drops, depending on age
Room sprays	1 teaspoon to 300ml (10fl oz) water
Wound washes	5–10 drops, depending on age, in 100ml ($3\frac{1}{3}$fl oz) water
Inhalations	2–5 drops, depending on age

Blending Small Proportions

The following gives the amount of essential oils to add in order to achieve 1, 2 or 3% dilution.

2 drops in 2 teaspoons ($\frac{1}{3}$fl oz) = approx 1%
4 drops in 2 teaspoons ($\frac{1}{3}$fl oz) = approx 2%
6 drops in 2 teaspoons ($\frac{1}{3}$fl oz) = approx 3%

Use dark coloured bottles to store the oils

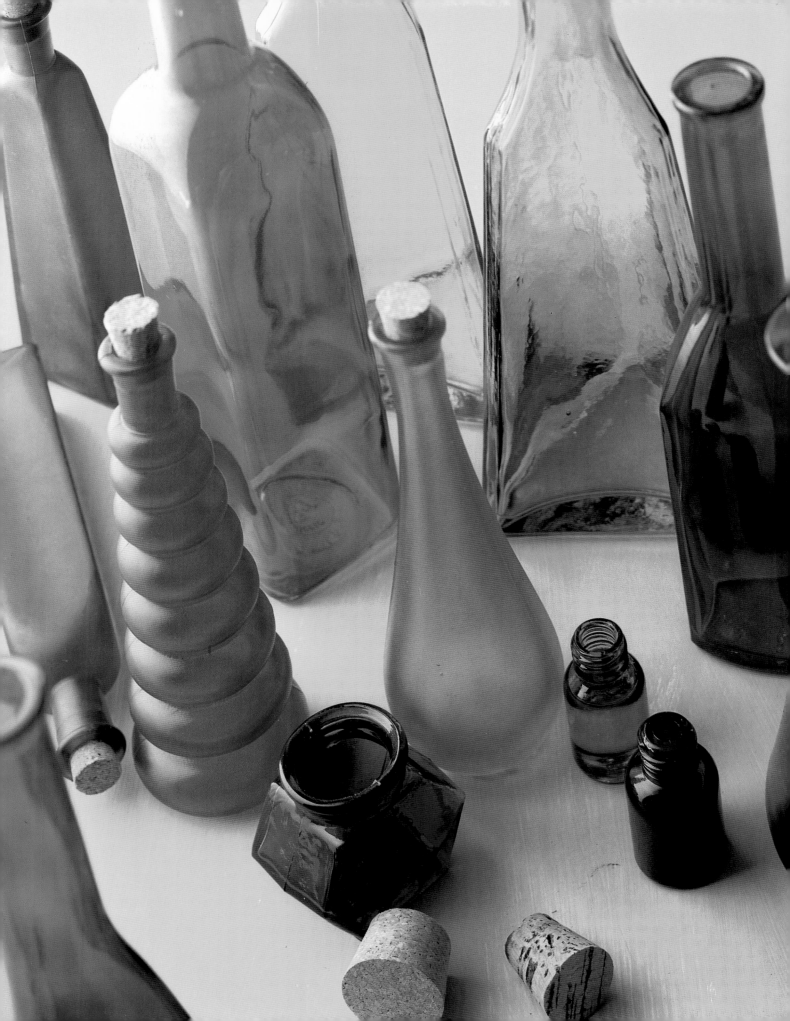

TIP

Air sprays are useful in all the rooms in the home. Use an antibacterial blend in the toilet, a relaxing blend in the bedroom, an invigorating and stimulating blend in the study/office and a soothing calming blend in the living and family rooms. You can create the atmosphere you desire by choosing appropriate blends.

Air Sprays

Antibacterial, antifungal and antiviral air sprays may be used to help prevent the spread of sickness, to relieve stress and insomnia and to deodorise the air. They are particularly useful in the toilet where they can be used to spray both the air and the surfaces, thus killing viruses and bacteria and helping to deodorise the area.

Air sprays are made by adding $\frac{1}{2}$–1 teaspoonful of essential oil(s) to 50ml ($1\frac{2}{3}$fl oz) of vodka or cider vinegar in a 300ml (10fl oz) pump spray bottle. Allow the ingredients to dissolve together, and then top up the bottle with purified water.

Baths

I love baths. I have a bath if I'm tired, if I'm stressed, if I'm happy, if I want to be alone—in fact, I will have a bath for any reason or no reason at all! Baths can fulfil many different functions and, depending on the water temperature and the oils used, they can be stimulating and bracing or relaxing and soothing. Baths which are too hot or too cold are not relaxing.

It is not generally realised that the skin, given optimum conditions, can be responsible for one-third of the excretion of waste matter from the body. By so doing, the liver, kidneys and lungs are relieved of quite a load. In order to work efficiently, the skin needs to be clean and free from dead cells which can block the pores. Using a body brush before bathing or showering helps to get rid of these dead cells.

If you do not have access to a bath, you can sprinkle a drop or two of the appropriate essential oil on a very wet flannel face cloth, partially wring it out and wipe it over your body. Another option is to make an air spray using oils for your particular problem—no more than 6 drops in a 200ml ($6\frac{1}{2}$fl oz) pump spray bottle. Shake the bottle well and spray your body lightly after you have finished washing, massage into your skin then pat dry.

Warm baths

The temperature for a relaxing bath should be about 27–34°C (80–93°F). Indulge for 20 minutes to … who knows how long?

Hot baths

The temperature for a bath to break a dry fever, increase perspiration and respiration and to eliminate toxins should be much hotter about 38–40°C (100–104°F), depending on what the patient can tolerate. The patient should remain in the bath for only about 10 minutes and be supervised constantly. After the bath, he or she should be wrapped in a warm towel, dried, helped into warm nightwear and into a warm bed. People with high blood pressure or heart problems should never have baths as hot as this.

Cold baths

The temperature for a cold bath should be between 21–27°C (70–80°F) for 2 to 5 minutes only. These baths (enjoyed by some Spartan characters!) improve breathing and muscle tone, decrease fatigue, improve thyroid function and skin tone, and often give relief from constipation.

Footbaths

Hot footbaths can be useful in staving off a cold or bout of 'flu if they are used as soon as the first symptoms appear. Alternating hot and cold footbaths can help to relieve a tension headache.

For a hot footbath, fill a bowl large enough for both feet with water as hot as can be tolerated. Sprinkle the appropriate essential oils on the surface of the water, mix thoroughly, and then immerse the feet. Soak for 10 to 15 minutes, topping up with more hot water as the temperature cools. (Take your feet out of the bowl before you add the water, or you might scald yourself.) Briskly rub the feet dry and put on some cosy footwear.

For a hot-and-cold footbath, fill 2 bowls (each large enough for 2 feet) with water, one cold and one as hot as can be borne. Sprinkle the appropriate oil on the surface of the cold footbath and mix well to disperse it. Soak the feet for a few minutes in the hot footbath and then in the cold one. Repeat this process for about 15 minutes.

TIP

With all aromatherapy bathing, the oils should be dripped into the bath after the water has been drawn. The water should then be thoroughly agitated to disperse the oils and so prevent any possibility of 'hot spots' or burns from the more powerful oils.

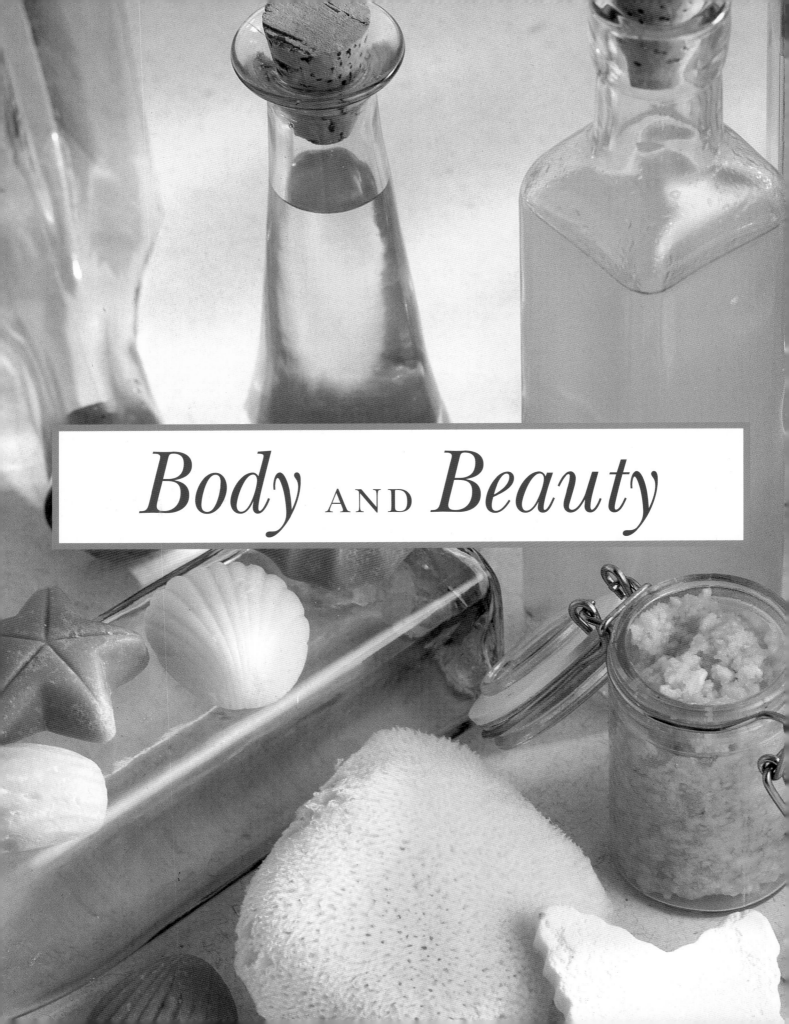

Body AND Beauty

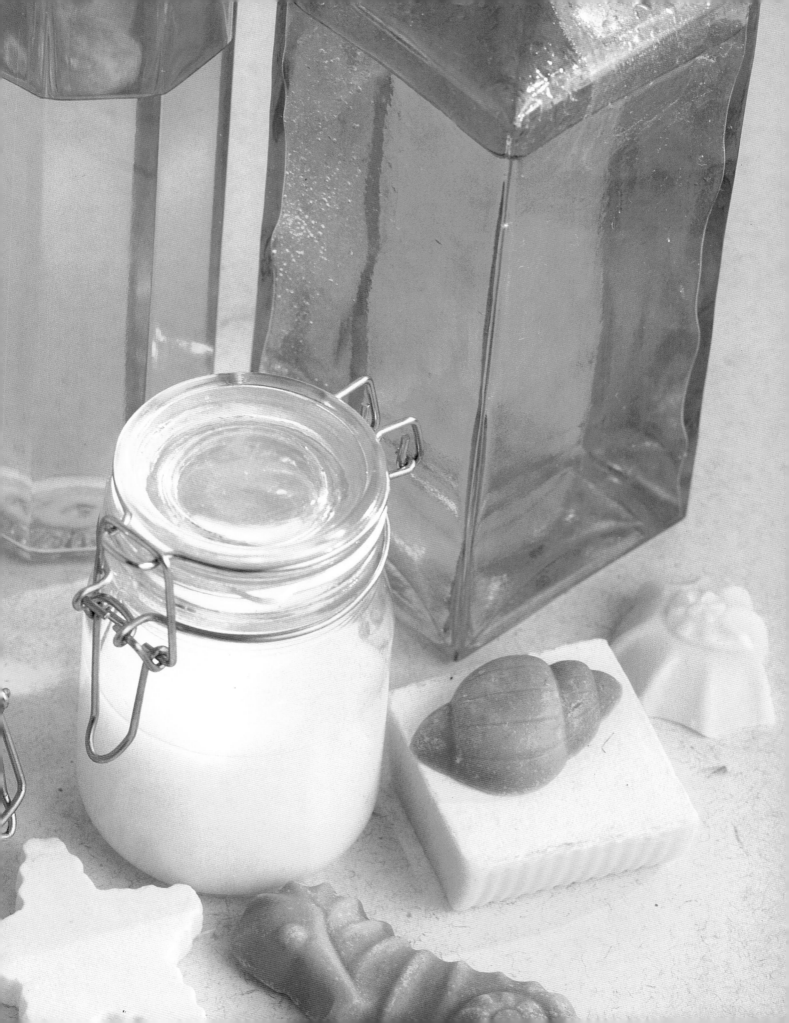

NOTE

Most commercial
skin and hair products
(particularly deodorants)
contain synthetic perfume;
this is because synthetics
are cheap and have a long
shelf life. These 'pretend'
oils have no therapeutic
or cosmetic value. In fact,
they can have a very
unpleasant effect on many
people, particularly
those who suffer from
allergic responses.

The Beauty of Home-made Products

Once you have begun to use essential oils on your hair and body, you will become aware of how synthetic the average commercial products do smell. I develop a quite painful ache inside my nose between my eyes whenever I visit the shampoo and cosmetics aisle in the supermarket and the odour from the various bottles and packets (particularly deodorants—yuk!) reaches my nose.

Home-made products which you can make using natural ingredients and pure essential oils will be a pure pleasure to your nose and will also benefit your body. I hope that you will enjoy making and using them as much as I do.

Proportions for Beauty Products

The essential oils must be measured very accurately as they are immensely powerful. If a recipe says to use 2 drops, then 4 drops will certainly not be better! Droppers or syringes and glass or plastic measures may be bought from pharmacies. The cautions and suggestions for quantities to use need to be carefully observed as the oils are immensely powerful. The difference in action between 1 and 2 drops is very great—1 drop of essential oil equals 1 cup of herbal infusion!

The following list is a general guide to amounts to use. Individual recipes may contain more or less essential oil.

Baths	4 to 10 drops maximum, depending on age
Compresses, facial	4 drops to 100ml ($3^{1}/_{3}$fl oz) water
Creams	10 to 15 drops in 50g (2oz) cream
Footbaths	4 to 6 drops, depending on age
Lotions	8 to 10 drops in 100ml ($3^{1}/_{3}$fl oz) liquid
Masks	2 drops in quantity for one mask
Massage oils	30 to 40 drops in 100ml ($3^{1}/_{3}$fl oz) carrier oil
Massage creams	20 to 30 drops in 50g ($1^{2}/_{3}$oz) cream

Hair Care

Many people spend an enormous amount of money during a year in their search for 'perfect' hair. What this is, I have not been able to quite work out: brunettes dye their hair red, redheads bemoan the fact that they are called 'carrots', blondes dye their hair brown, grey hair becomes ash, and curly hair becomes straight while straight hair goes curly!

Television advertisements show girls with huge manes of supposedly 'perfect' hair which tosses wildly in what must be the full force of a wind machine. If it has not already happened, these same young women look as though they are going to suffer from dislocated necks, due to the violent head movements they make to show us what we can expect if we use the same brand of shampoo and conditioner as they do. Well ... I do not believe a word of it.

Your hair type is, largely, genetically predisposed, and if you have fine, limp hair or prematurely thinning hair you can probably look to your parents to see where you inherited it from.

The following pages contain many lovely treatments which will add natural body and shine to dry hair, control grease and dandruff and gently and fragrantly care for all hair types. Essential oils can also help to repair damage and keep coloured, bleached or dyed hair in good condition.

TIP

Essential oils can help repair damage hair and keep coloured, bleached or dyed hair in good condition

Essential Oils for Hair

General Hair Care	Cedarwood, clary sage, geranium, lavender, rosemary
Dry Hair	Geranium, lavender, rosemary, sandalwood
Oily Hair	Clary sage, cypress, lavender, lemon, rosemary
Normal Hair	Lavender, lemon, geranium, rosemary
Dandruff	Cedarwood, clary sage, lavender, rosemary, sandalwood.
Fragile Hair	Chamomile, clary sage, lavender, sandalwood
Loss of Hair	Cedarwood, juniper, lemon, rosemary
Scalp Tonic	Cedarwood, chamomile, clary sage, lemon, rosemary, tea tree, ylang-ylang
Split Ends	Rosewood, sandalwood

Pre-shampoo Treatments

Wash mitt from Crabtree & Evelyn, flowers from Lisa Milasas

If your hair is naturally dry or has become dry due to over-shampooing, bleaching, colouring, or too much sun or illness, both hair and scalp will benefit from a hot oil treatment.

Hot Oil Treatment

2 tablespoons castor oil
1 tablespoon olive oil
10 drops lavender oil
5 drops clary sage oil
5 drops sandalwood oil

Mix all the oils together and warm to blood heat (no hotter). Massage into the hair and scalp. Cover hair with a piece of towelling wrung out in very hot water, and then with a shower cap. Wrap the whole head in a hot towel. Reheat this towel when it cools. Repeat a few times, and do not shampoo for at least an hour. Follow with a herbal shampoo. The quantities in this recipe may need to be doubled if your hair is very long or thick.

Egg and Honey Treatment

For dry, damaged or fine hair
1 egg yolk, beaten
2 teaspoons castor oil
1 teaspoon runny honey
dried milk powder, to mix
2 drops sandalwood oil
2 drops clary sage oil

Mix the first three ingredients together; add enough dried milk to make a paste. Add the essential oils and mix well. Rub the paste thoroughly into the hair and scalp. Cover the hair with a plastic shower cap and then wrap the whole head in a hot towel. Alternatively, wrap the head in a towel wrung out in very hot water. Leave for 20 minutes. Shampoo with a mild herbal shampoo.

Ingredients for making
pre-shampoo treatments

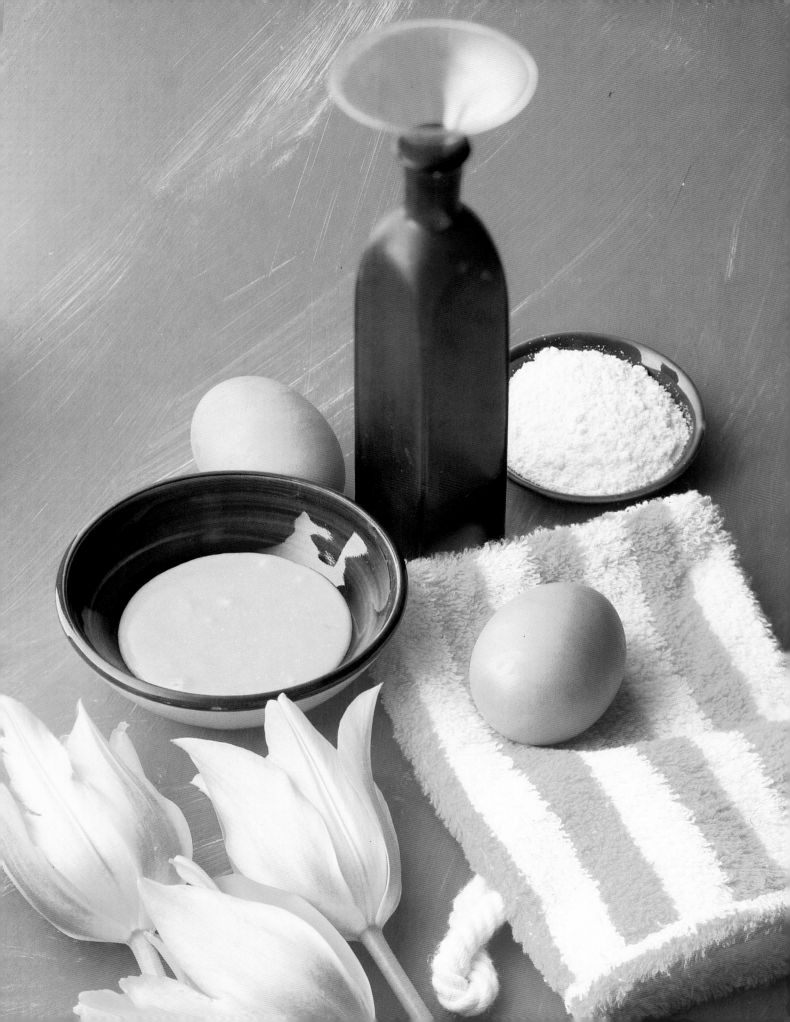

TIP

Detergent based
shampoo strips hair of its
natural oil and that is why
wax conditioners are
needed.
These conditioners
only coat the hair giving
the illusion of shine
and health.

'Real' Shampoos, Rinses and Dressings

Many shampoos claim to be 'herbal', but if you read the list of contents you will usually find the herbal content is at or near the bottom. This means that this ingredient is only contained in the smallest amount possible. It does not matter how little there is of a herb or herbal extract, the product may still legally be called 'herbal'. (This applies to creams, lotions and many other preparations as well.)

Commercial shampoos are, basically, the same formula as carpet shampoo. One of the main ingredients is a foaming agent. We have been conditioned to believe that seeing plenty of foam means that the product is cleaning well, when in fact the foam has nothing to do with the product's cleaning capacity—it is purely for our gratification.

Add essential oils to the best shampoo you can find; the most wholesome are often to be purchased in health food stores. Try diluting the shampoo half and half with water. You will be astonished to find that it cleans just as well, is far gentler on your hair and has cost you half the price. The essential oils may be added to the bottle of shampoo after it has been diluted, but they need to be very well blended. Alternatively, you can add the oils to a tablespoon of shampoo just before washing your hair.

Detergent-based shampoo strips the hair of all its natural oil and that is why wax conditioners are needed. The following recipe is for a natural herbal shampoo based on soap. This is the type of shampoo our grandmothers used before the advent of detergents. Their hair was certainly no worse than ours and, frankly, I think that it was much better. Soap-based shampoo will not strip your hair of its natural oils, but you will need to use an acid rinse afterwards as soap is alkaline.

At first, using this herbal shampoo may feel completely different from your regular purchased brands, but persevere—your hair and hip pocket will both thank you! After about three weeks (it takes this long to get rid of wax conditioners, fillers and other chemical ingredients from the hair shafts) you will really begin to enjoy your new hair treatment.

Basic Herbal Shampoo

80–100g (approx. 3oz) pure soap flakes, or the same
amount of bar soap, finely grated
1 litre (32fl oz) hot water
2 teaspoons borax
30–40 drops single or mixed essential oils
(choose from the Essential Oils for Hair list)

Stir soap, water and borax together until completely dissolved. Reheat if necessary. Cool. Add the blended oils or single essential oil of choice. Stir thoroughly until completely incorporated. This shampoo may go lumpy after standing. It does not matter—just give it a good stir until it is blended again.

After-shampoo Rinse

500ml (16fl oz) cider vinegar
2 teaspoons mixed or single essential oils
(choose from the Essential Oils for Hair list)

Mix all the ingredients together in a 500ml (16fl oz) bottle. Leave for 4 days to blend.
To use: Add ½ cup (125ml/4fl oz) of the rinse to 1 litre (32fl oz) of warm water. Rinse the hair, using a bowl to catch the drips. Repeat rinsing as often as you like, or until your arms are too tired.

Hair Dressing

A hair dressing is used between shampoos to keep hair glossy, smooth and healthy. The non-greasy essential oils are absorbed into the hair shaft, making it suitable for all hair types.

2 teaspoons lavender oil
2 teaspoons rosemary oil
½ teaspoon geranium oil
½ teaspoon jojoba oil (for dry or damaged hair only), or
½ teaspoon juniper oil (for other hair types)

Mix all the ingredients together in a 25ml (approx. 1fl oz) dark-coloured dropper bottle.
To use: Put a few drops in the palm of one hand and then rub your hands together. Now, rub your palms through your hair. This treatment can be used as often as you like.

Towel from Sheridan, flowers from Lisa Milasas

Skin Care

Essential Oils for Skin

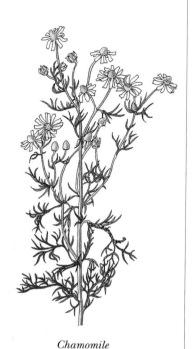

Chamomile

Benzoin

Styrax benzoin

COSMETIC USES: Antiseptic. Reduces inflammation of the skin. Helps to clear fungal infections of the skin and skin irritations. Makes the skin more elastic. Good for cracked and dry skin, particularly on hands and feet. Extends the shelf life of cosmetic preparations. Excellent in perfumes as a fixative.

Chamomile, German and Roman

Anthemis nobilis, Matricaria chamomilla

COSMETIC USES: Reduces puffiness and inflammation. Improves elasticity in ageing skin. Non-irritating for sensitive skin. May help to heal acne, dermatitis, eczema, thread veins.

Frankincense

Boswellia thurifera, B. carterii

COSMETIC USES: Revitalises dry and ageing skin. May help to prevent or reduce wrinkles. A good gentle 'balancer' for oily skin.
CAUTION: Can be irritating if used directly on the skin.

Geranium

Pelargonium odoratissima and other species

COSMETIC USES: An 'all-rounder', good for cleansing and toning all skin types. Brings an improved flow of blood to the skin, thus helping to heal problems such as acne, dermatitis and eczema.

Jasmine

Jasminum officinale

COSMETIC USES: Useful for all skin types as it softens and smooths. Particularly good for dry, sensitive skin. One of the important perfume oils.

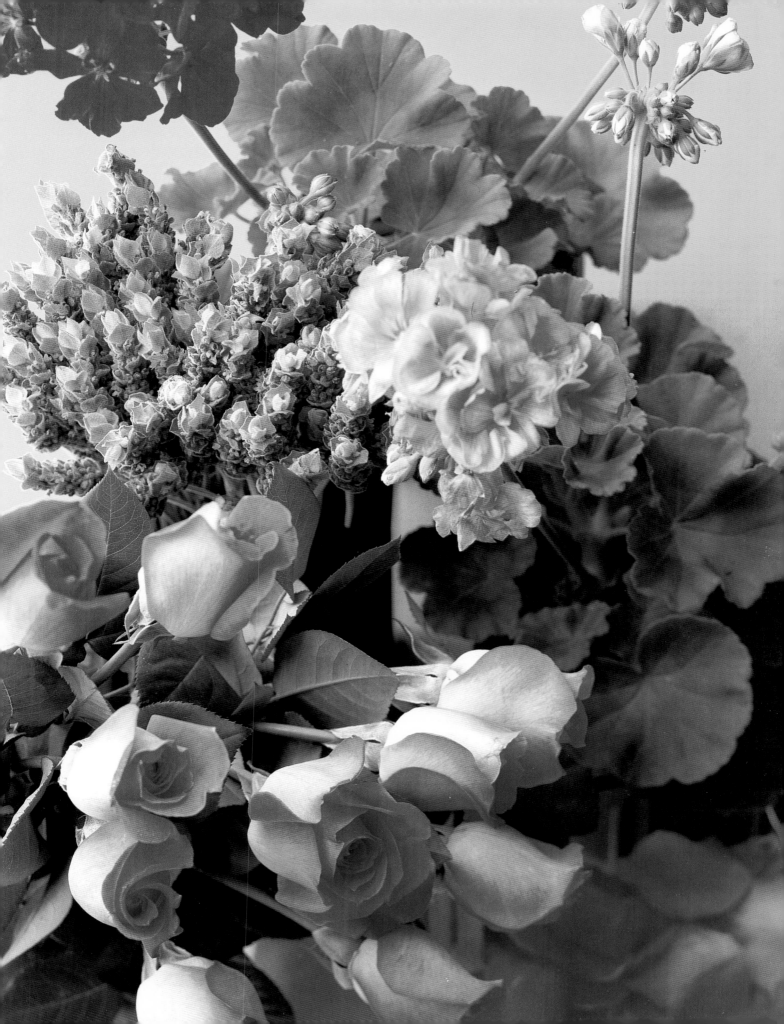

Juniper

Juniperus communis

COSMETIC USES: One of the most useful oils for clearing an oily skin and scalp. Its antiseptic and purifying properties make it useful for aiding in the healing of acne, dermatitis and eczema. May also be used in cellulite treatments.
CAUTION: Not to be used during pregnancy.

Lavender

Lavandula angustifolia, L. officinalis

COSMETIC USES: A most valuable oil for all skin types as it balances sebum and promotes the growth of new cells. Particularly useful for mature skin and wrinkles. It has proved to be helpful when treating acne, dermatitis, eczema and pimples. Useful as a deodorant, and a very good insect repellent. May be used in treatments for thread veins.

Lemon

Citrus limonum

COSMETIC USES: Cleanses and brightens oily skin and hair. Softens scar tissue. Strengthens brittle nails. Helps to remove dead skin cells. Useful in the treatment of acne.

Neroli (Orange Blossom)

Citrus vulgaris

COSMETIC USES: Useful for all skin types, but particularly for sensitive, dry and mature skin. Has a reputation for being a cell proliferant and also for improving skin elasticity. Has deodorant properties; also used widely in perfumes. Used in treatments for thread veins.

Palmarosa

Cymbopogon martinii

COSMETIC USES: One of the most valuable skin oils. Restores water balance, stimulates cell growth, regulates sebum production. Has a reputation for delaying the appearance of wrinkles and softening those which have already appeared. Aids in the treatment of acne, dermatitis, eczema, psoriasis and other skin problems.

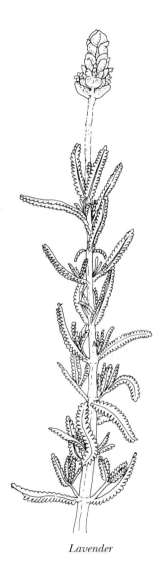

Lavender

Patchouli

Pogostemon cablin

COSMETIC USES: Useful in the treatment of skin disorders, inflammation, fungal infections, dandruff and scalp disorders. Good for treating oily skin and hair, open pores and wrinkles. Used in perfumery as a fixative and to give a sensuous, earthy 'bottom note'.

Rose

Rosa centifolia, R. damascena, R. gallica

COSMETIC USES: All skin types, particularly dry, inflamed, mature and sensitive skin. Useful for treating broken capillaries, skin allergies and wrinkles.

Rosewood

Aniba roseaodora

COSMETIC USES: Excellent for general skin care; suitable for sensitive, combination, oily and dry skin types. Useful for treating scars, wrinkles and thread veins. A 'cell regenerator'.

Sandalwood

Santalum album

COSMETIC USES: Useful for dry, ageing and dehydrated skin conditions, especially crepey skin on throats, eczema and cracked or chapped skin. Also helpful for treating inflammation, itching and acne.

Ylang-Ylang

Cananga odorata

COSMETIC USES: For general skin care, particularly for irritated and oily skin conditions and ageing skin.

NOTE

It is comforting to know that you can deal with simple problems by swift and appropriate action. It is beyond the scope of this book to deal with serious complaints and it must always be borne in mind that seemingly simple symptoms may mark serious ailments. Seek professional help if a condition persists or worsens.

Which Oils to Use Where?

Here is a guide to the different essential oils to use for various skin conditions. Choose a blend of oils suited to your skin type.

ACNE	Chamomile, geranium, juniper, lavender, palmarosa, patchouli, sandalwood
AGEING SKIN	Frankincense, rose, neroli, ylang-ylang
ALLERGIES	Chamomile
ALL SKIN TYPES	Geranium, jasmine, lavender, neroli, palmarosa, rose, rosewood
ANTISEPTIC	All essential oils, to some degree, especially benzoin, geranium, lavender, juniper
ASTRINGENT	Benzoin, geranium, juniper, lemon, patchouli, rose, sandalwood
BALANCER	Frankincense, geranium
CELL GROWTH	Frankincense, geranium, lavender, neroli, palmarosa, rose
CELLULITE	Juniper, lemon
CRACKED, DRY SKIN	Benzoin, sandalwood
DEHYDRATED SKIN	Sandalwood
DEODORANT	Benzoin, bergamot, cypress, geranium, lavender, neroli, patchouli, rosewood
DERMATITIS	See Acne
DRY SKIN	Jasmine, rose, rosewood, palmarosa, lavender, sandalwood
ECZEMA	Chamomile, geranium, juniper, lavender, palmarosa
ELASTICITY	Benzoin, chamomile, neroli

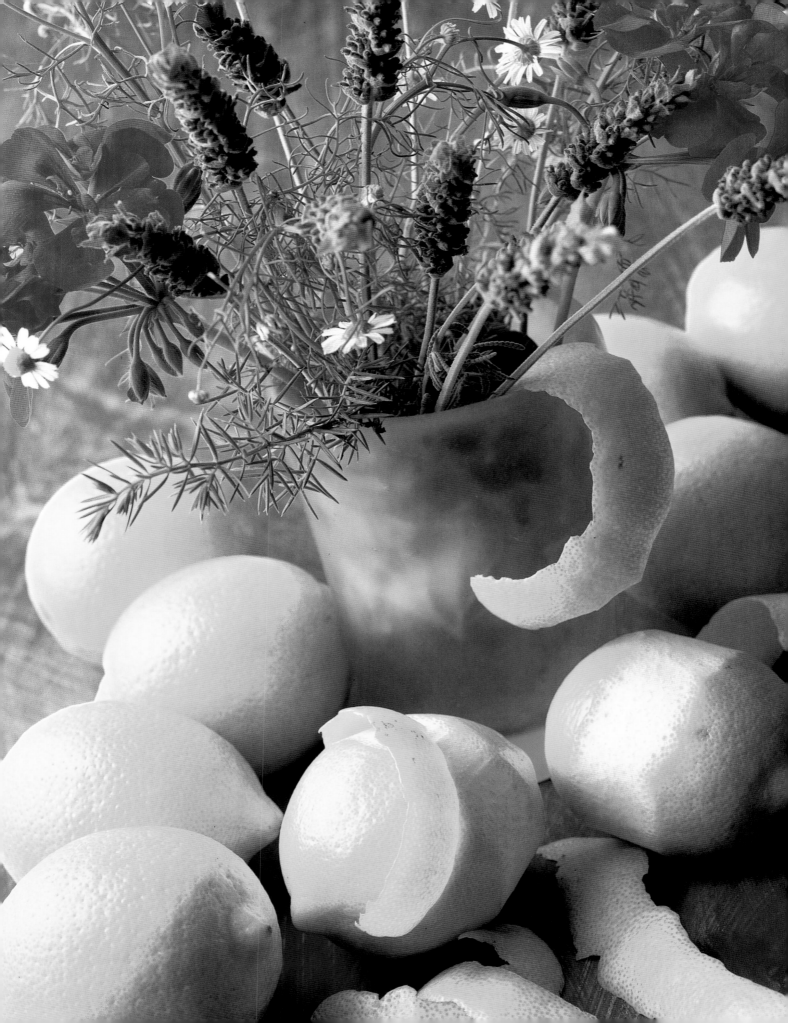

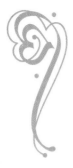

EMOLLIENT	Chamomile, geranium, jasmine, lavender, rose, sandalwood
FIXATIVE (perfume)	Benzoin, patchouli
FUNGAL INFECTIONS	Benzoin, patchouli
INFLAMMATION	Benzoin, chamomile, rose, sandalwood
MATURE SKIN	Lavender, neroli, rose
NORMAL SKIN	Geranium, lavender, jasmine, neroli, palmarosa, rose, rosewood, ylang-ylang
OILY SKIN	Juniper, lemon, patchouli, rosewood, ylang-ylang
PRESERVATIVE	Benzoin
PUFFINESS	Chamomile, geranium, rose
SCARS	Chamomile, frankincense, geranium, juniper, lavender, lemon, patchouli, rosewood
SEBUM	Regulator palmarosa
SENSITIVE SKIN	Chamomile, jasmine, neroli, rose
THREAD VEINS	Chamomile, lavender, lemon, neroli, rose, rosewood.
WRINKLES	Frankincense, lavender, palmarosa, patchouli, rose, rosewood

Vegetable Oils

Vegetable oils are used to act as 'carrier' oils for the essential oils. Some of the best are apricot kernel, avocado, canola, grapeseed, olive, safflower, sweet almond and wheat germ oils. Cold-pressed oils are the best to use as they still retain antioxidants, and therefore remain fresh for much longer. They also seem to retain a much larger amount of vitamins and minerals. Suitable carrier oils will be suggested in each section.

Facial Treatments

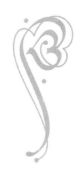

As babies, we usually have perfect skin: smooth, close-textured, moist, and with enough oil to protect but not cause problems. As we get older, hormonal changes, heredity factors and the ageing process all begin to change the texture of our skin. We need to know how to care for our individual skin type in order to keep it looking as good as possible for as long as possible.

Following are recipes and treatments for every type of skin. If you do not have the essential oils listed in a particular recipe, they may be changed by consulting the list of Which Oils to Use Where? and choosing other oils with similar properties.

The recipes are suitable for both men and women. Men suffer from skin problems just as often as women do, but it is usually assumed that men 'just have skin'. In the recipes where the fragrance lingers on the skin I have suggested different oils for men, as the perfume of some of the oils might be perceived as 'too feminine'.

Carrier Oils

APRICOT OIL	A light non-drying/semi-drying oil suitable for all skins.
AVOCADO OIL	A beautiful thick green semi-drying oil invaluable in moisture creams and lotions.
CANOLA OIL	A non-drying oil excellent in massage oils and in creams and lotions for dry and normal skins.
GRAPESEED OIL	A fine, semi-drying oil suitable for most skins. Very good basic carrier as it is light, clean and has no smell.
OLIVE OIL	A rich non-drying oil excellent formassage oils, creams, soaps and lotionsfor dry and normal skins.
SAFFLOWER OIL	A semi-drying polyunsaturated oil and excellent all-rounder.
SWEET ALMOND OIL	A fine, emollient, non-drying oil for all skin types.
WHEAT GERM OIL	A nourishing, fine, healing oil.

Steaming

Facial steaming causes the skin to perspire, which in turn helps to loosen grime, dead skin cells and hardened sebum. The heat increases the blood supply to the surface of the skin and also hydrates it, giving a more youthful, softer skin tone with a clearer, brighter colour.

If thread veins are a problem, you will need to be very careful when steaming. Apply a thick layer of moisturiser or night cream over the veined area and hold your face about 40cm (16in) away from the steam—no closer. Do not steam your face more than once a fortnight.

People with normal, oily and combination skin types may use facial steaming as often as twice a week, if liked.

Steaming Instructions

Have ready a shower cap, a large towel and a heat-proof pad for the table.

1. Wash or cleanse the face. Put the shower cap on.
2. Place 2 litres (64fl oz) of boiling water in a bowl; set the bowl on a heat-proof, non-slip mat on the table.
3. Drop 2 drops of essential oil or 1 teaspoon of one of the following blends onto the surface of the water. Quickly form a tent with the towel over the bowl and your head.
4. Keep your face about 20cm (8in) away from the steam, close your eyes and enjoy the facial steam for about 5 to 10 minutes.
5. Splash your face with cool (not cold) water and finish with a face tonic and some moisturising cream.

The following blends make a sufficient amount for about ten steaming treatments.

Normal and Combination Skin

8 drops geranium oil
6 drops palmarosa oil
4 drops ylang-ylang or lavender oil
3 tablespoons sweet almond oil

Mix all the ingredients together in a 60ml (2fl oz) bottle. Shake well to mix, and also shake before each use. Store in a cool, dark place, but do not refrigerate. Use 1 teaspoonful of the mixture for each facial steam treatment.

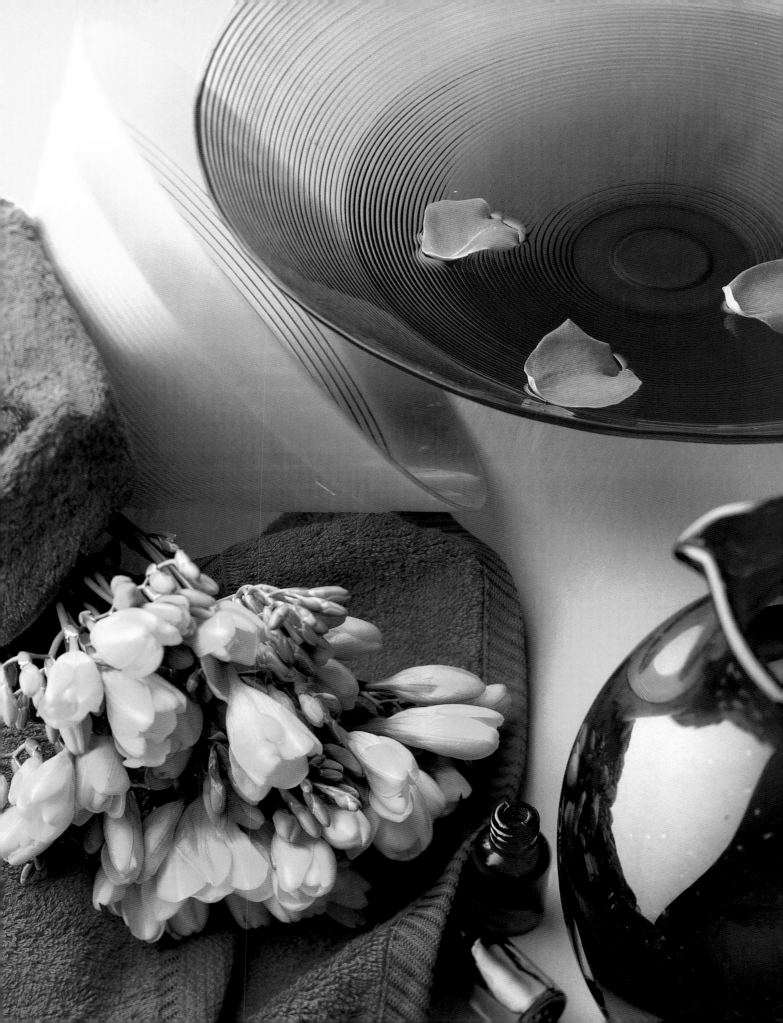

The frequency with which you use scrubs depends on your skin type. If you have oily blemished skin, you can use these preparations several times a week but if your skin is fine and dry, choose only the most gentle treatment and use it maybe once a fortnight.

Dry Skin

8 drops rosewood oil
6 drops palmarosa oil
4 drops rose or lavender oil
3 tablespoons sweet almond oil

Mix the ingredients in a 60ml (2fl oz) bottle. Shake well and also shake before use. Store in a cool, dark place—do not refrigerate. Use 1 teaspoonful of the mixture for each facial steam treatment.

Oily Skin

12 drops lemon oil
4 drops patchouli oil
2 drops sandalwood oil
3 tablespoons vegetable oil

Mix the ingredients in a 60ml (2fl oz) bottle. Shake well and also shake before use. Store in a cool, dark place—do not refrigerate. Use 1 teaspoonful of the mixture for each facial steam treatment.

Ageing and Mature Skin

12 drops chamomile oil
4 drops frankincense oil
2 drops lavender or rose oil
3 tablespoons vegetable oil

Mix the ingredients in a 60ml (2fl oz) bottle. Shake well and also shake before use. Store in a cool, dark place—do not refrigerate. Use 1 teaspoonful of the mixture for each facial steam treatment.

Acne, Eczema and Problem Skin

8 drops juniper oil
4 drops geranium oil
6 drops lavender oil
3 tablespoons vegetable oil

Mix the ingredients in a 60ml (2fl oz) bottle. Shake well and also shake before use. Store in a cool, dark place—do not refrigerate. Use 1 teaspoonful of the mixture for each facial steam treatment.

Scrubs

Scrubs exfoliate the skin, meaning they clear excessive oiliness, refine the pores, improve circulation and generally nourish the skin. They leave the skin looking fresh and rosy. Scrubs should never be used on thread veins, as they would stimulate the area and possibly aggravate the condition. Scrubs are best suited to normal, combination and oily skin types.

Almond and Rosewood Scrub

For Normal and Combination Skin

This scrub may be made suitable for dry skin types by using orange juice instead of the cider vinegar and adding one teaspoon of honey to the mixture.

2 teaspoons sweet almond oil
1 tablespoon very finely ground blanched almonds
1 teaspoon cider vinegar
2 drops rosewood oil
purified water

Mix all the ingredients, adding sufficient water to form a paste. Massage gently into the skin of the face and throat, rinse with lukewarm water and pat dry. Apply moisturising cream or lotion.

Yeast and Yoghurt Scrub

For Oily, Normal and Combination Skin

Yeast stimulates the circulation, bringing blood to the surface of the skin. When using this scrub, be very careful not to over-stimulate the cheeks where the capillaries are delicate and near the surface. Those with thread veins should avoid using this scrub.

1 tablespoon yoghurt
2 teaspoons almond meal
1 teaspoon brewer's yeast
1 teaspoon runny honey
1 drop geranium oil
1 drop lemon oil

Mix all the ingredients together to form a paste. Massage gently into the skin of the face and throat, rinse off with lukewarm water and pat dry. Apply moisturising cream or lotion.

TIP

Masks can be most

pleasurable and beneficial

beauty treatments. They

can help to rejuvenate,

cleanse, soothe and hydrate

the skin, and they also help

to prevent wrinkles. Masks

may be used with benefit by

all skin types, but should

not be used over areas

where thread veins are

present.

Masks

With each of the following recipes, spread the mask mixture over your face and neck. Lie down with pads of cottonwool soaked in distilled witch hazel or cooled chamomile tea over your eyes. Relax for 10 to 15 minutes—and enjoy! Wash the mask off in lukewarm water, followed by a splash of cool water.

Kaolin and Orange Mask

For Normal Skin

1 egg, beaten
1 teaspoon olive oil
2 teaspoons orange juice
1 teaspoon honey
1 drop rose or geranium oil
1 drop rosewood or jasmine oil
dried milk powder, to mix

Mix all the ingredients together, adding just enough dried milk powder to make a smooth paste.

Golden Glow Mask

For Dry Skin

1 egg yolk, beaten
1 teaspoon olive oil
2 teaspoons orange juice
1 teaspoon honey
1 drop carrot oil (optional)
2 drops neroli or geranium oil
dried milk powder, to mix

Mix all the ingredients together, adding just enough dried milk powder to make a smooth paste.

A selection of prepared
masks ready to apply

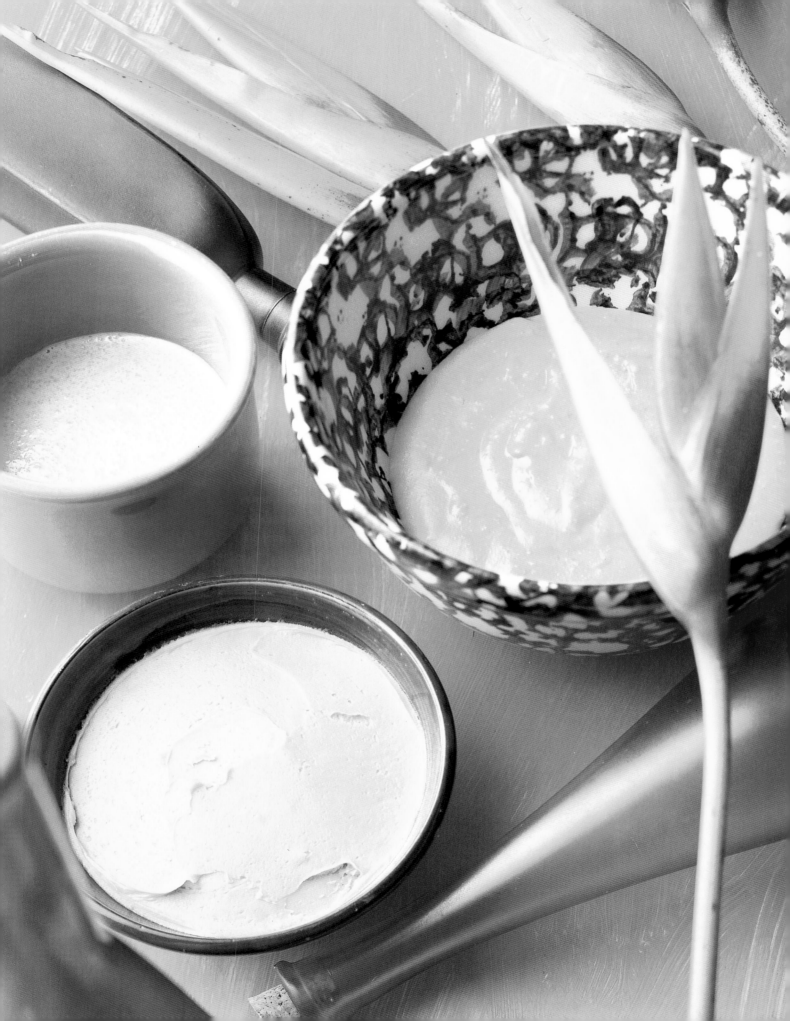

Face masks can also be made with finely grated fresh fruit mixed with essential oils. Pawpaw (papaya) and cucumber are both excellent for the face. You can mix in a little kaolin clay powder to thicken the pulp a little. Choose essential oils suitable for your skin type—you will only need a drop or two of the oils.

Yeast and Yoghurt Mask

For Oily and Combination Skin
1 tablespoon brewer's yeast
1½ teaspoons yoghurt
1 teaspoon distilled witch hazel
1 teaspoon olive oil
1 teaspoon wheat germ oil
1 drop palmarosa oil
1 drop lemon oil
finely ground rolled oats or kaolin clay powder
(from the pharmacy), to mix

Mix all the ingredients together, using just enough rolled oats or kaolin to make a soft paste.

Egg and Almond Mask

For Sensitive Skin
1 egg yolk, beaten
1 teaspoon jojoba oil
½ teaspoon honey
1 drop chamomile oil
1 drop carrot oil
1 teaspoon powdered milk or cornflour
water or rose-water, to mix

Combine the egg yolk, jojoba oil, honey and essential oils in a small bowl. Add the powdered milk or cornflour and mix well. Add enough water or rose-water to make a smooth paste.

Healing Mask

For Acne, Eczema and other Skin Problems
1 tablespoon finely ground almonds
2 teaspoons cornflour or kaolin clay
1 teaspoon honey
1 drop juniper oil
1 drop chamomile oil
1 drop lavender oil
water, to mix

Mix all the ingredients together, adding enough water to the mixture to form a soft paste.

Cleansers

Daily cleansing is possibly the most important part of your skin care routine. Your face is subjected to oily fumes from traffic, dust, synthetic cosmetics and many other things which clog the skin's pores and make it look dull and lifeless.

Washing Waters

Special washing water may be used to cleanse the face if the skin is very sensitive, or if it is troubled with acne, pimples or other skin problems. It may also be used as a moisturising lotion with the addition of one teaspoonful of sweet almond oil or other fine-textured oil. Shake mixture vigorously to blend the oil before use.

50ml (2fl oz) rose-water
50ml (2fl oz) purified water, less 1 teaspoon
$^{1}/_{4}$–$^{1}/_{2}$ teaspoon glycerine (try the $^{1}/_{4}$ first, and increase if you like it)
6 drops essential oil (choose a suitable blend from the list of
Which Oils to Use Where?)

Mix all ingredients together in a 100ml ($3^{1}/_{3}$fl oz) bottle. Shake well to blend thoroughly. Leave for 4 days, shaking occasionally. Filter mixture through coffee filter paper. Store in a dark-coloured glass bottle. Shake well before use.

TO USE: take a palm-sized piece of cottonwool, dip it in warm water and squeeze out well. Flatten it out into a pad, sprinkle with the washing water and use to cleanse throat and face. Repeat if necessary. There is no need to use a toner after this treatment.

Cleansing Cream

For Dry, Ageing and Sensitive Skin

These skin types usually feel very uncomfortable if they are treated with soap and water. I have dry skin and I have not used soap and water on my face for about 40 years!

A cleanser for dry, ageing and sensitive skin needs to be gentle. The following recipe is simple, inexpensive and pleasant to use. It should not be refrigerated and will need to be made fresh every two weeks or so. If copha is not available in your area, there is sure to be a similar solid vegetable cooking fat. This recipe can be adapted to the thickness you prefer by changing the amount of olive or canola oil.

TIP

Cleanse your skin with one of the home-made cleanser products each day following the instructions for your particular skin type. If you have dry, ageing or sensitive skin, treat it with great care as it is not as robust as an oily, normal or combination skin type.

TIP

The essential oils in the Glycerine and Honey Soap recipe are just suggestions—choose whichever scent you like best. If you suffer from acne or pimples, you could add 10 drops of tea tree oil and reduce the quantity of rosemary oil to 20 drops.

Cleansing Cream

1 tablespoon olive or sweet almond oil
60g (2oz) copha (hydrogenated coconut oil solid cooking fat)
1 drop benzoin oil (optional)
10 drops rosewood oil
10 drops palmarosa oil (sandalwood for men)

Melt the olive or canola oil and copha together in a small bowl over a pan of boiling water. When melted, remove from the heat and beat until mixture has cooled to blood heat. Add the benzoin oil and the essential oils and beat until well incorporated. Pot up in a clean glass jar. Refrigerate only if the weather is very hot.

Glycerine and Honey Soap

Those of you with normal, combination and oily skin types may prefer to use soap to cleanse your face and neck. The following soap is simple to make and gives the benefits of essential oils, glycerine and honey, plus it has a yummy natural smell unlike most commercial soaps. The glycerine and honey are both humectants, which means that they attract moisture to the skin and hold it there.

2–3 tablespoons water
$4^{1}/_{2}$ cups (550g/1lb 2oz) finely grated unscented pure soap
2 teaspoons glycerine
2 teaspoons honey
30 drops rosemary oil
10 drops lavender oil

Microwave the water and soap on HIGH (100% power) for 2 to 3 minutes until bubbly, scrape down and stir after 1 minute. If it is too thick, add more water and reheat. Use the least water possible, or the soap will shrink a lot as it dries. Add the glycerine and honey and keep stirring until they are completely incorporated. Add the essential oils when the mixture has cooled slightly.

Press the soap into moulds (such as soap dishes, individual jelly moulds, milk cartons cut in half, little baskets lined with muslin), or shape it into balls. Set aside in an airy place to dry for 2 to 6 weeks. When the soap is hardened, you may like to polish it. Lightly moisten a cloth with some water to which a drop or two of essential oil has been added, and then buff the soap.

Glycerine and Honey
Soap in the making

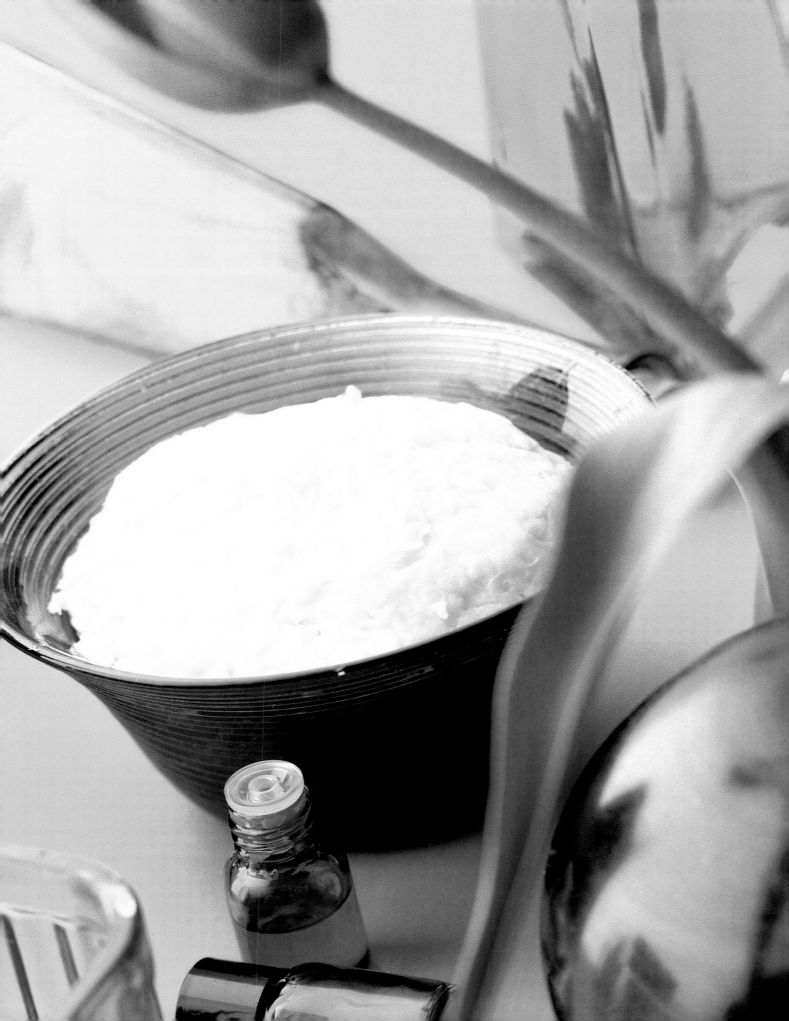

TIP

To use toners and astringents, moisten a piece of cottonwool in water, squeeze out all excess moisture and flatten it to a pad. Pour a little toner or astringent on this pad and wipe it gently over the face and throat to remove any surplus cleanser.

Toners and astringents remove surplus oil from the skin, gently stimulate the circulation, restore the skin's acid mantle and leave it feeling fresh and clean. Toners which contain alcohol or a large amount of distilled witch hazel are called astringents and they should not be used on dry, sensitive or ageing skin. Even very oily skin types should avoid too-frequent applications of astringents containing a lot of alcohol, as this stimulates the oil glands.

Toners and astringents may also be used to remove makeup, or as a freshener during the day.

'Magic Three' Toner

For Acne and Troubled Skin

½ cup (125ml/4fl oz) rose-water
¼ cup (60ml/2fl oz) purified water
1 teaspoon cider vinegar
5 drops juniper oil
3 drops sandalwood oil
2 drops chamomile oil
¼–½ teaspoon glycerine

Mix all the ingredients together in a bottle. Shake well to blend. Allow mixture to mature for a few days, shaking occasionally.

'Top of the Morning' Astringent or Aftershave

For Oily and Combination Skin

½ cup (125ml/4fl oz) distilled witch hazel
¼ cup (60ml/2fl oz) purified water
1 tablespoon cider vinegar
5 drops sandalwood oil
3 drops benzoin oil
2 drops spearmint oil
¼–½ teaspoon glycerine

Mix all the ingredients together in a bottle. Shake well to blend. Allow mixture to mature for a few days, shaking occasionally.

Gentle Rose Toner

For Dry and Ageing Skin
$^3/_4$ cup (200ml/6$^1/_2$fl oz) rose-water
$^1/_4$ cup (60ml/2fl oz) purified water
3 drops rosewood or rose oil
3 drops palmarosa oil
$^1/_2$ teaspoon glycerine

Mix all the ingredients together in a bottle. Shake well to blend. Allow mixture to mature for a few days, shaking occasionally.

Lavender Witch Hazel Toner

For Normal and Combination Skin
$^1/_4$ cup (60ml/2fl oz) rose-water
$^1/_2$ cup (125ml/4fl oz) distilled witch hazel
$^1/_4$ cup (60ml/2fl oz) purified water
10 drops lavender oil
$^1/_4$ teaspoon glycerine

Mix all the ingredients together in a bottle. Shake well to blend. Allow mixture to mature for a few days, shaking occasionally.

Sunrise Aftershave

For Normal and Combination Skin
The following aftershave is gentle, but very thorough. It helps to contract the skin after shaving without drying it out.

$^3/_4$ cup (200ml/6$^1/_2$fl oz) distilled witch hazel
$^1/_4$ cup (60ml/2fl oz) purified water
5 drops sandalwood oil
3 drops benzoin oil
2 drops rosemary oil
$^1/_4$ teaspoon glycerine

Mix all the ingredients together in a bottle. Shake well to blend. Allow mixture to mature for a few days, shaking occasionally.

TIP

Aftershaves are much stronger than toners and are more suited to oily or combination skins.

Moisturising Oils

In order to introduce moisture to the skin we need to use both oil and water. Used alone, water evaporates—but when it is used in combination with oil, the water is held on the skin until it is massaged in.

Primrose Path Moisturising Oil

For Dry Skin
40ml (1$\frac{1}{3}$fl oz) sweet almond oil
40ml (1$\frac{1}{3}$fl oz) olive oil
1 teaspoon avocado oil
1 teaspoon wheat germ oil
60 drops evening primrose oil
10 drops jojoba oil
5 drops carrot oil
10 drops palmarosa oil (sandalwood for men)
5 drops rosewood oil
5 drops lavender oil
2 drops sandalwood oil (benzoin for men)
2 drops patchouli oil (neroli or frankincense for men)

Place all ingredients in a 100ml (3$\frac{1}{3}$fl oz) bottle. Shake well for several minutes. Leave for 4 days to blend. Store in a dark, cool place. Shake before use.

Dew Drops Moisturising Oil

For Normal and Combination Skin
$\frac{1}{3}$ cup (90ml/3fl oz) sweet almond oil
1 teaspoon avocado oil
1 teaspoon wheat germ oil
30 drops evening primrose oil
10 drops jojoba oil
5 drops carrot oil
10 drops palmarosa oil (sandalwood for men)
5 drops rosewood oil
5 drops geranium oil (benzoin for men)
5 drops ylang-ylang oil (neroli or frankincense for men)

Place all the ingredients in a 100ml (3$\frac{1}{3}$fl oz) bottle. Shake well for several minutes. Leave for 4 days to blend. Store in a dark, cool place. Shake before use.

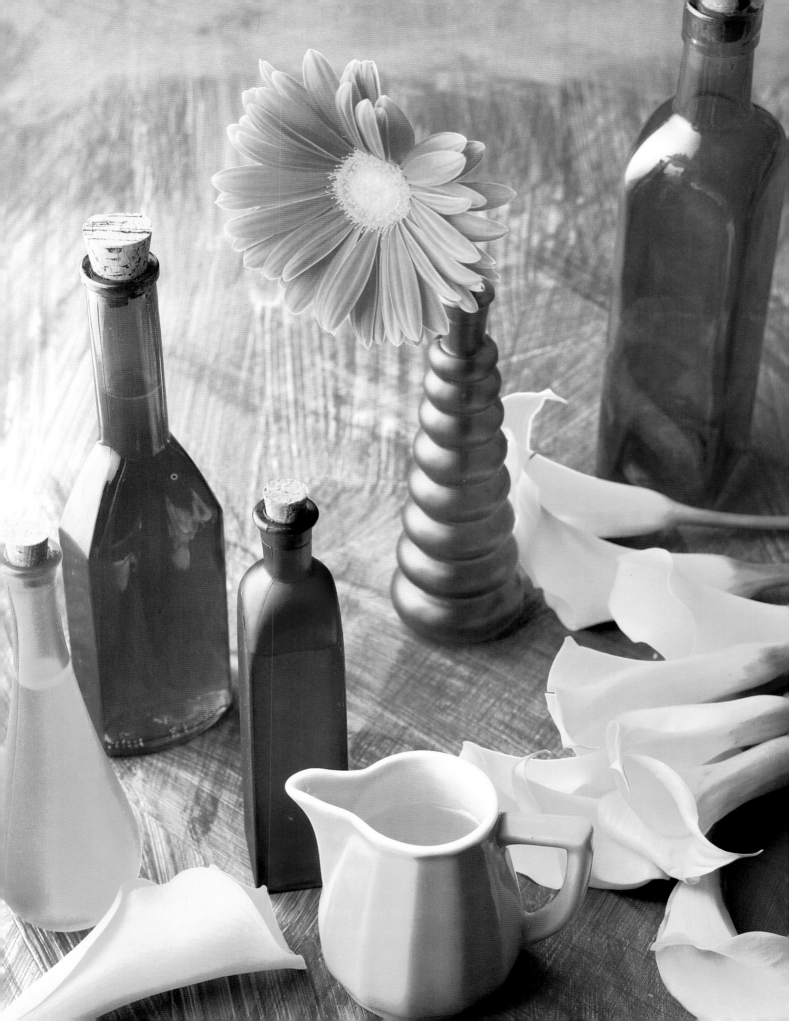

TIP

Mineral water sprays are lovely and cooling on a hot day if they are kept in the refrigerator until used. Spray a little on the face and throat, then apply a few drops only of a moisturising oil and gently smooth it into the skin until it is absorbed. You will find that this treatment feels far less heavy than the application of some creams, particularly during warm weather.

Satin Skin Gel

For Oily, Combination and Normal Skin

Those of you with oily skin can count yourselves fortunate, because your skin will wrinkle much less and more slowly than other skin types. The following gel makes a lovely oil-free treatment.

100g (about 3¹/₃oz) 95% or 100% aloe vera gel
25 drops of mixed essential oils (see Silk Skin Moisture Oil)

Add the oils to the gel and mix very well. Blending might take a little time and needs to be done very thoroughly.

Silk Skin Moisturising Oil

For Oily Skin

Use this oil on the throat, around the eyes and the lips and also apply a thin smear of it over the whole face last thing at night.

¹/₃ cup (90ml/3fl oz) grapeseed oil
50 drops evening primrose oil
40 drops carrot oil
10 drops lemon oil
10 drops lavender oil
5 drops juniper oil

Place ingredients in a 100ml (3¹/₃fl oz) bottle. Shake well. Leave for 4 days. Store in a dark, cool place. Shake before use.

Apricot and Avocado Moisturising Oil

For Sensitive Skin

This blend contains only the gentlest oils. Nevertheless, test all the oils on your skin before using on your face.

¹/₃ cup (90ml/3fl oz) apricot kernel oil
60 drops evening primrose oil
40 drops wheat germ oil
5 drops chamomile oil
5 drops rosewood or rose oil
2 drops lavender or neroli oil

Place ingredients in a 100ml (3¹/₃fl oz) bottle. Shake well. Leave for 4 days to blend. Store in a dark, cool place. Shake before use.

Under-eye Oil

Fragile, thin and easily damaged: this describes the skin under our eyes. Use only the gentlest and most precious oils on this delicate area. First moisten the skin around and under the eyes. Then pat a few drops of the oil onto the skin, using the middle finger of your right hand (left if you are left-handed). This is the weakest finger and so it exerts the least pressure. Keep patting gently to help the oil to be absorbed. Leave for 20 minutes and then blot off any surplus oil. Do not allow the oil to go in your eyes as it might sting.

2 x 250IU vitamin E capsules
1 tablespoon sweet almond oil
1 teaspoon jojoba oil
20 drops evening primrose oil
4 drops palmarosa oil

Pierce the capsules and mix the contents with the other oils in a 25ml (approx. 1 fl oz) dark glass bottle. Shake well. Leave 4 days, shaking often. Store in a dry, dark, cool place. Do not refrigerate.

'Most Precious' Night Oil

This extremely rich and luxurious oil is suitable for all skin types. The essential oils will help to regulate and balance the sebum content, and to smooth, soothe and soften the skin. Spray or splash the skin lightly with water then apply a few drops of this oil.

2 teaspoons sweet almond oil
$1^1/_2$ teaspoons apricot kernel oil
1 teaspoon hazelnut or grapeseed oil
$1^1/_2$ teaspoons olive oil
1 teaspoon jojoba oil
1 teaspoon avocado oil
1 teaspoon wheat germ oil
5 drops evening primrose oil
5 drops carrot oil
5 drops palmarosa oil
5 drops rosewood or rose oil
5 drops geranium oil
5 drops ylang-ylang or jasmine oil

Mix the ingredients in a 60ml (2fl oz) bottle. Shake well. Leave for 4 days to blend. Keep in a dark, cool cupboard. Do not refrigerate.

When applying any of the moisturising oils in these pages, massage into the skin gently using just the fingertips and not the palm of the hands. Always stroke softly in an upward direction (gravity is intent on dragging us down—we don't need to give it any assistance!).

Oral Care

When we are young we are invincible. We are confident that we will keep our teeth until the day we die. We crack nuts, remove bottle tops (I'm cringing as I write!) and break tough cotton thread with our teeth. We forget to floss, eat sweets between meals and generally treat them in a very cavalier fashion.

It is hopefully never too late to change our ways, and the following recipes will help to ensure the health of teeth and gums. The toothpowder recipe is also good for cleaning dentures—you still need to care for them and for your gums.

Toothpowder

½ cup (125g/4oz) fine sea salt
½ cup (125g/4oz) soda bicarbonate
8 drops peppermint oil
5 drops lemon oil
2 drops myrrh oil

Mix the sea salt and soda bicarbonate very well. Add the mixed essential oils very slowly, a drop at a time, stirring constantly to prevent the mixture from lumping. Keep in separate jars.

Mouthwash

A mouthwash is used to help to sweeten the breath, and to heal sores, ulcers and gum problems. If bad breath is an ongoing problem it would be wise to look for the source of the problem. A visit to the dentist may be needed or, if the cause is a digestive one, eating 1–2 cups daily of yoghurt which contains both acidophilus and bifidus cultures will create a healthier digestive system.

⅓ cup (90ml/3fl oz) cider vinegar
1 tablespoon brandy
1 teaspoon glycerine
10 drops peppermint oil
10 drops lemon oil
5 drops myrrh oil

Pour all the ingredients into a 100ml (3⅓fl oz) glass bottle. Stand for 4 days, shaking occasionally. Strain. Store in a dark cupboard.
TO USE: Add 1 teaspoonful to ¼ cup (60ml/2fl oz) of warm water. Rinse mouth thoroughly with mixture, but do not swallow it.

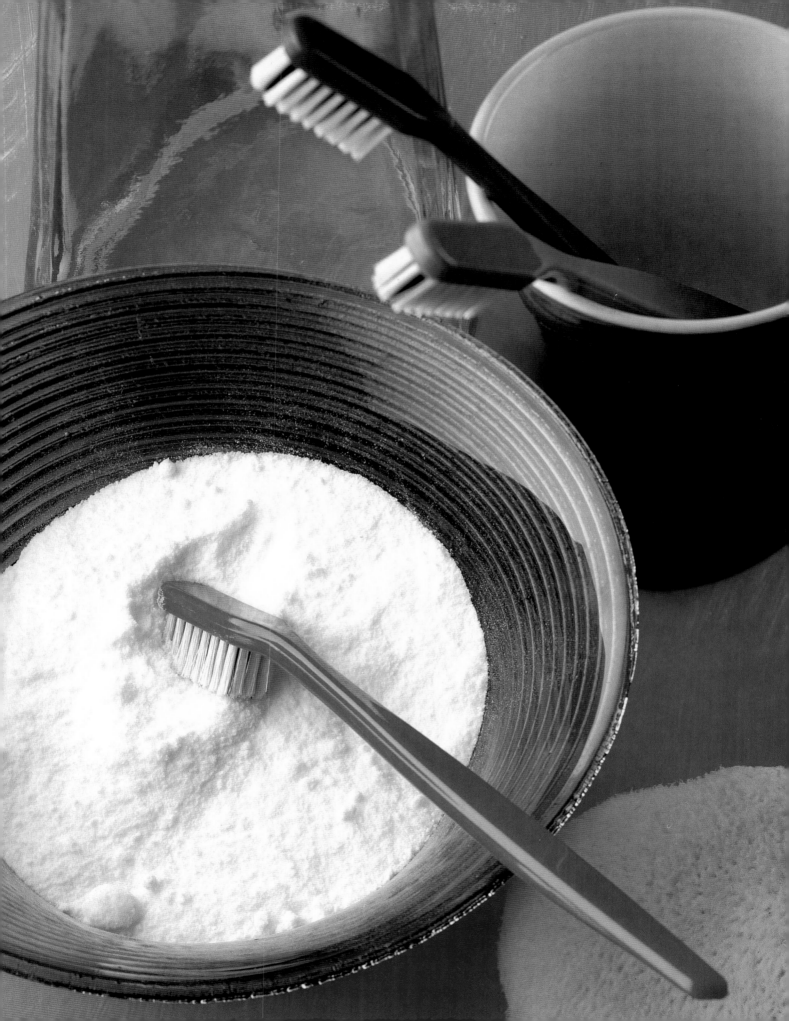

Lips should always be
kissable but unfortunately
are often dry, cracked or
plagued with cold sores.
You can use the Lip Salve
(at right) both at night and
during the day.

Lip Salve

Lips have much thinner, drier skin than the rest of the face. Dry, cracked lips can be painful and unsightly. Regular use of the following lip salve will help to keep the skin soft and moist. If you do not use lipstick, carry a little pot of this lip salve in your pocket or handbag, and use it often during the day.

15g (½oz) beeswax
1 teaspoon anhydrous lanolin
1 tablespoon wheat germ oil
3 tablespoons olive oil
1 teaspoon glycerine
2 x 250IU vitamin E capsules
10 drops jojoba oil (optional)
20 drops lemon oil

Melt the beeswax and lanolin in a jar or small bowl over a pan of boiling water. Stir in the wheat germ and olive oils, and then remove the mixture from the heat. Beat in the glycerine until no free drops of glycerine are apparent. When mixture has cooled a little, pierce the vitamin E capsules, squeeze in the contents and then add the remaining oils. Mix thoroughly. Pot up in small clean glass jars with tight-fitting lids.

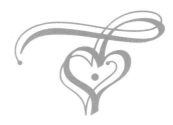

The Neck

The skin on the neck is usually much drier than that on our faces, and it is often very neglected, resulting in a crepey, dry texture. The following oil blend is gentle and rich. If used regularly, it can help to keep wrinkles at bay and to soften and smooth those which have already appeared.

'Neck Special' Anti-wrinkle Oil

2 x 250 IU vitamin E capsules
2 teaspoons jojoba oil
1 teaspoon avocado oil
1 teaspoon wheat germ oil
½ teaspoon evening primrose oil
5 drops carrot oil
5 drops lavender oil
5 drops palmarosa oil
5 drops rosewood oil

Pierce the vitamin E capsules and mix the contents with all the other oils in a 25ml (approx. 1fl oz) dark-coloured glass bottle. Shake well to mix. Leave for a few days to blend, shaking often. Store in a dry, dark, cool place. Do not refrigerate.

To USE: Spray or splash a little water on the throat. Sprinkle a few drops of the oil onto the palm of your hand and massage gently into the throat in an upwards direction until it has been absorbed.

TIP

When applying oils or creams to the neck area, always apply gently in an upward motion to encourage the skin to stay firm and toned.

TIP

Try to become accustomed to using gloves when working or, if you really hate rubber gloves, use the Lavender Barrier Cream before starting a dirty job. Get into the habit of massaging the Healing Hand Cream into your hands after you wash them and before bedtime.

It is very common to spend a great deal of time and money on our hair and faces, and to neglect our poor hands. They are exposed to the weather just as our faces are, and they also have to contend with gardening, washing clothes and dishes and all the other jobs which are so hard on skin.

Lavender Barrier Cream

1 tablespoon purified water
2 tablespoons olive oil
2 teaspoons kaolin clay powder (from the pharmacy)
10 drops lavender oil
*10 drops *simple tincture of benzoin (from the pharmacy)*

Mix all the ingredients together thoroughly. Pot up in a clean glass jar. Massage cream well into hands before doing dirty jobs.
* NOTE: Do not confuse this with compound tincture of benzoin (Friar's Balsam). It contains other ingredients and is not suitable for this recipe.

Healing Hand Cream

If you do not have the time or energy to make a cream from scratch, the following recipe is for you. The aloe cream and essential oils will heal and soften sore, dry or cracked skin. Buy the aloe cream from a health food store, making sure you get one containing the largest amount possible of aloe.

50g (2oz) jar aloe cream
1/2 teaspoon benzoin oil
10 drops sandalwood oil
10 drops palmarosa or lavender oil
10 drops lavender oil

Decant the cream into a small bowl. Mix the oils together and add slowly to the cream, a drop at a time, mixing constantly. When the oils are thoroughly incorporated, spoon the cream back into the jar. Use it after washing your hands and at bedtime.

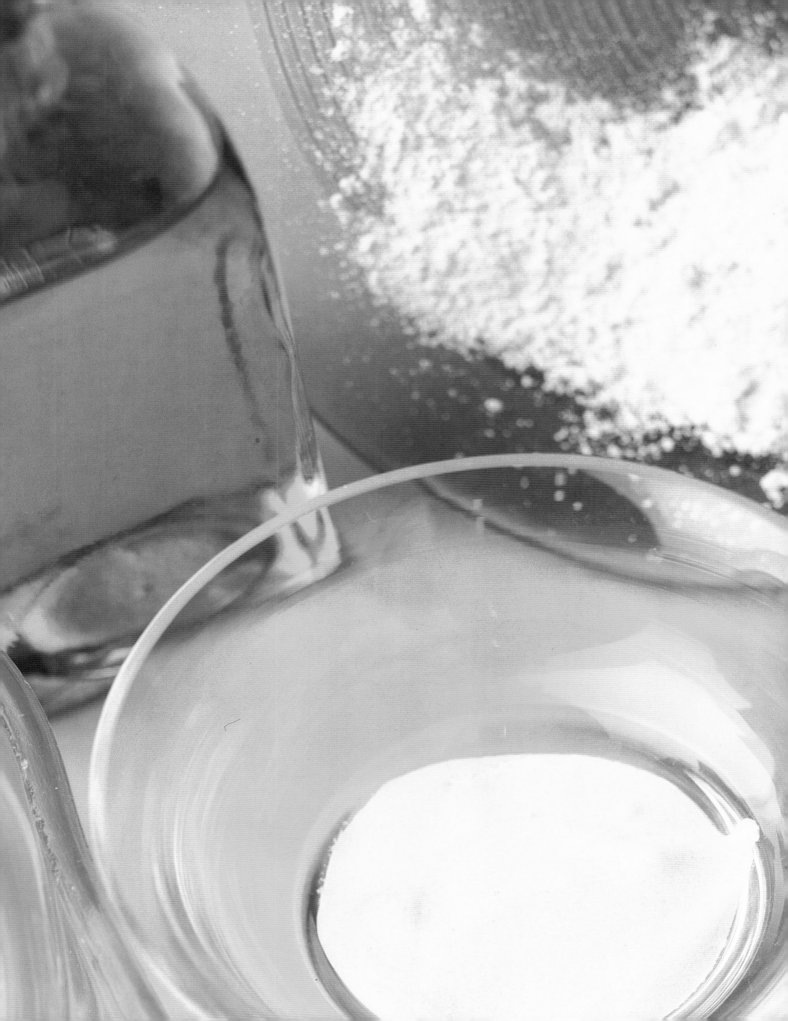

When your feet become
tired from walking;
standing at work or
shopping; from sports; and
from general running
around, try having the hot
and cold footbath
described in the Foot Relief
Bath, followed by a massage
using 6 to 8 drops of the
luxuriant Foot-ease Oil for
each foot.
Your feet will sigh with
relief and respond quickly
to this treat.

Hand and Nail Oil

4 x 250 IU vitamin E capsules
1 tablespoon almond oil
2 teaspoon avocado oil
2 teaspoon olive oil
1 teaspoon jojoba oil
20 drops evening primrose oil
5 drops benzoin oil
10 drops sandalwood oil
10 drops lemon oil

Prick the vitamin E capsules and squeeze the contents into a 60ml (2fl oz) bottle. Add all the other oils and shake well to blend. Leave for 4 days before use, shaking often.

To use: Pour 4 to 6 drops into the palm of your hand. Massage oil into the skin and around the nail bed until absorbed. Repeat.

The Feet

Foot Relief Bath

Fill 2 bowls (each to fit 2 feet) with water—one cold and one as hot as can be borne. Sprinkle 4 to 6 drops of rosemary or lavender oil or 2 to 3 drops of each oil in the cold footbath and agitate well to disperse the oil. Soak the feet for a few minutes first in the hot footbath, and then in the cold. Repeat for about 15 minutes.

Foot-ease Oil

1 tablespoon almond oil
2 teaspoons avocado oil
1 teaspoon wheat germ oil
2 teaspoons jojoba oil
10 drops rosemary oil
10 drops lavender oil
5 drops benzoin oil
1 teaspoon vodka

Mix all the ingredients in a 60ml (2fl oz) bottle. Shake well. Leave for 4 days to blend, shaking often.

Baths and Body Oils

There are few people who do not enjoy a bath. I think that one of the reasons we find baths so relaxing is that the water gets rid of all the prickly positive ions which make us feel so stressed and tired. Even just a short bath (perish the thought!) is better than no bath at all. If you do not feel comfortable with the idea of taking your dirt into the bath and soaking in it, then you can have a quick shower first.

Have the bathroom at a comfortable temperature and place all your bathtime goodies within easy reach. Use a bath pillow or a hot water bottle full of warm water on which to rest your head. The rest is up to you ... candles, incense, music, books, a drink, big fluffy towels will all enhance this pleasurable experience. Add 5 to 10 drops of essential oil to the water after the bath has been drawn. Agitate the water to disperse the oils thoroughly. The temperature for a relaxing bath should be 27–34°C (80–93°F). Indulge for half an hour, or as long as you can get away with it. And don't forget to put a notice on the door saying 'Please do not disturb'!

Basic Semi-dispersible Bath Oil

This oil will almost disperse in the bath water. Vodka is expensive, but as this recipe makes enough for about 30 baths, each luxury bath becomes extremely affordable. My personal choice, cider vinegar, adds its own distinctive aroma to the oils and also has the benefits of being inexpensive and therapeutic.

1/2 cup (125ml/4fl oz) vodka or cider vinegar
2 tablespoons good quality shampoo
3 teaspoons glycerine
3 teaspoons essential oils (see Bath Oil Blends which follow)

Mix all the ingredients together in a bottle. Invert several times to mix well. Leave for 4 days to blend, inverting several times again. Add 1½ teaspoons of the mixture to the water after the bath has been drawn. Agitate the water to disperse the mixture thoroughly. Lean back and enjoy!

TIP

If you do not have access to a bath (what possessed you to buy or rent a house without one?!) you can sprinkle a drop or two of the appropriate essential oil on a very wet flannel face cloth, partially wring it out and then wipe it over your body after a shower. Another option is to make an air spray using essential oils for your particular needs—no more than 6 drops in a 200ml (6½fl oz) pump-spray bottle. Shake the bottle well and spray your body lightly after you have finished washing. Massage the oils into your skin. Pat dry with a towel.

Soap dishes from Dinosaur Designs, towel from Sheridan

Bath Oil Blends

With all the following suggested essential oil blends, mix the oils together in a tiny bottle and leave for 4 days before adding to the Basic Semi-dispersible Bath Oil recipe. Shake during the 4 days.

Children

$^1/_2$ teaspoon chamomile oil
$^1/_2$ teaspoon lavender oil
$^1/_2$ teaspoon geranium oil

Normal Skin

1 teaspoon geranium oil
1 teaspoon rosewood oil
1 teaspoon ylang-ylang oil

Dry Skin

1 teaspoon lavender oil
1 teaspoon rosewood or rose oil
1 teaspoon palmarosa oil

Oily Skin

$^1/_2$ teaspoon juniper oil
2 teaspoons lemon oil
$^1/_2$ teaspoon patchouli oil

Itchy Skin

$^1/_2$ teaspoon chamomile oil
$^1/_2$ teaspoon juniper oil
$^1/_2$ teaspoon lavender oil
1 teaspoon sandalwood oil

Sleep Well

$^1/_2$ teaspoon chamomile
1 teaspoon lavender oil
1 teaspoon marjoram oil
$^1/_2$ teaspoon sandalwood oil

Anti-cellulite

2 teaspoons juniper oil
1 teaspoon lemon oil

Colognes

I enjoy using colognes more than concentrated perfumes, as they can be sprayed or splashed liberally onto the body to create an 'aura' of scent without being overpowering.

Some of the essential oils in the following blends will not be found in the list of Essential Oils for Skin Care as they are not actually skin oils; they are, however, necessary to create a beautifully balanced perfume.

Colognes are a blend of 60 parts alcohol, 15 parts purified water, 5 parts glycerine and 15 parts essential oil(s). Vodka is the best alcohol to use as it has no smell. The glycerine gives 'body' to the blend and counteracts the drying effect of the alcohol. These parts, if converted to quantities, are as follows in the basic blend.

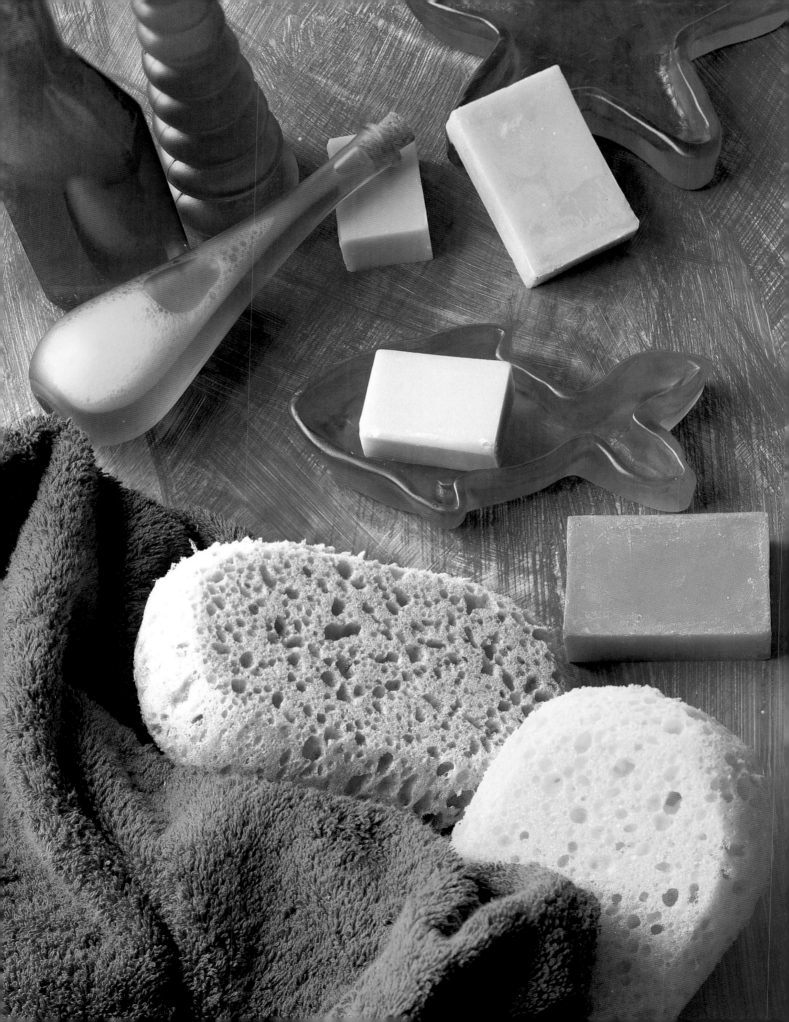

NOTE

The strength of perspiration odour seems to be determined by many factors: puberty or hormonal changes, high intake of meat, junk food, alcohol and stress. Clothing made of synthetic fabric does not allow the body to breath and the perspiration to evaporate and this compounds the problem.

Basic Cologne Blend

2 tablespoons vodka
2 teaspoons purified water
$^1/_4$ teaspoon glycerine
$1^1/_2$ teaspoons essential oil

With all the following recipes, mix all the ingredients together in a 60ml (2fl oz) bottle. Shake well and leave for between 2 to 6 months to mature. The initial scent will bear little resemblance to the final perfume, so patience is needed.

Flower Garden

$^1/_2$ teaspoon bergamot oil
$^1/_2$ teaspoon geranium oil
20 drops petitgrain or neroli oil
20 drops palmarosa oil

Sweetheart

1 teaspoon rosewood oil
10 drops jasmine oil
20 drops ylang-ylang oil
10 drops bergamot oil

Macho Man

1 teaspoon sandalwood oil
30 drops cedarwood oil
10 drops rosewood oil
5 drops lemon oil

Enticement

1 teaspoon ylang-ylang oil
15 drops patchouli oil
15 drops sandalwood oil
5 drops jasmine oil
5 drops rose oil

Lavender Lady

$1^1/_2$ teaspoons lavender oil
10 drops lemon oil
10 drops palmarosa oil

Deodorants

There are only a few areas of the body where the smell of perspiration is a problem: these are the feet and armpits. The sweat glands in these areas are different from those found elsewhere on the body, and they produce more profuse and stronger-smelling sweat. Fresh perspiration does not smell, but it decomposes very rapidly and so becomes really unpleasant.

The following recipe is for a light deodorant which is very pleasant and quite safe to use. The smell of the vinegar vanishes in a very short time, leaving only the scent of the essential oils.

Fresh-as-a-Daisy Deodorant—For Her

100ml ($3^{1}/_{3}$fl oz) cider vinegar
100ml ($3^{1}/_{3}$fl oz) witch hazel
20 drops bergamot oil
20 drops lavender oil
10 drops patchouli oil
10 drops rosewood oil
10 drops benzoin oil
$^{1}/_{2}$ teaspoon glycerine

Combine the ingredients in a bottle and shake well. Leave for 4 days, shaking occasionally. Store in a dark, dry, cool place.
To use: Splash or spray on after showering, and as needed.

Forest Fantasy Deodorant—For Him

100ml ($3^{1}/_{3}$fl oz) cider vinegar
100ml ($3^{1}/_{3}$fl oz) witch hazel
20 drops benzoin oil
20 drops bergamot oil
20 drops cypress oil
5 drops rosewood oil
10 drops eucalyptus oil
$^{1}/_{2}$ teaspoon glycerine

Combinethe ingredients in a bottle and shake well. Leave for 4 days, shaking occasionally. Store in a dark, dry, cool place.
To use: Splash or spray on after showering, and as needed during the day.

Deodorant Powder

6 tablespoons unperfumed talcum powder
6 tablespoons cornflour
20 drops lavender oil
20 drops myrrh oil
10 drops patchouli oil
5 drops lemon oil

Sieve the powder and cornflour together in a bowl. Mix the essential oils together. Add the oil mixture, a drop at a time, to the powder mixture, stirring constantly to prevent the powder from going lumpy. Store in an airtight container.

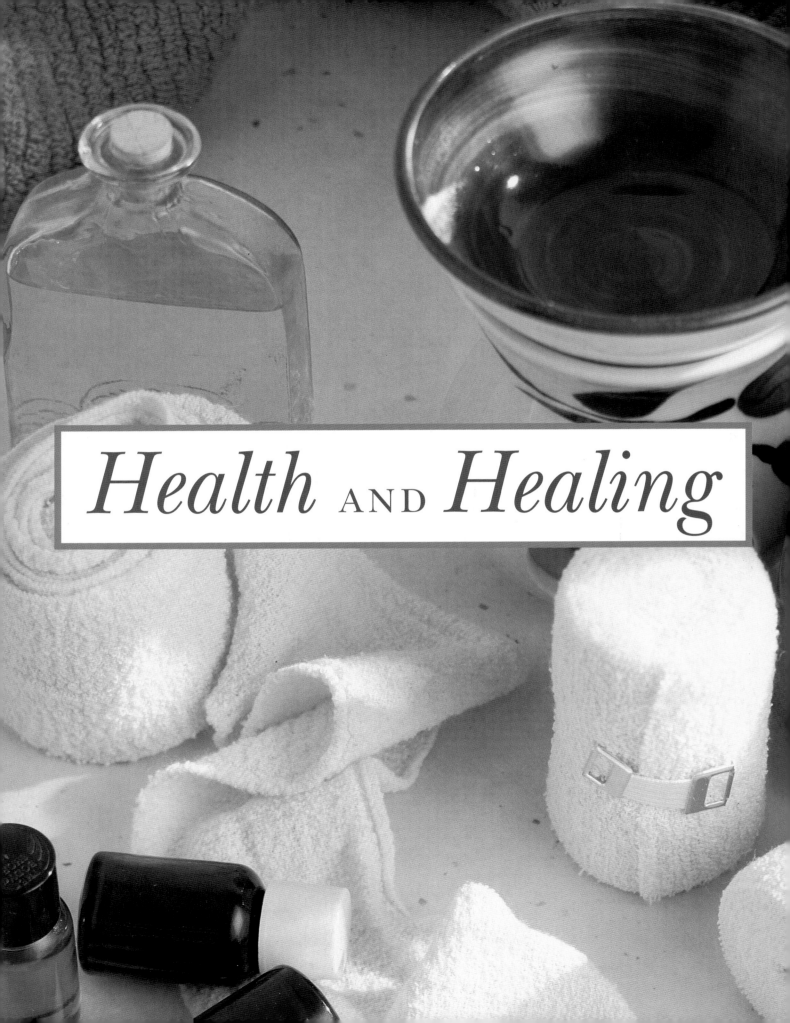

Health AND Healing

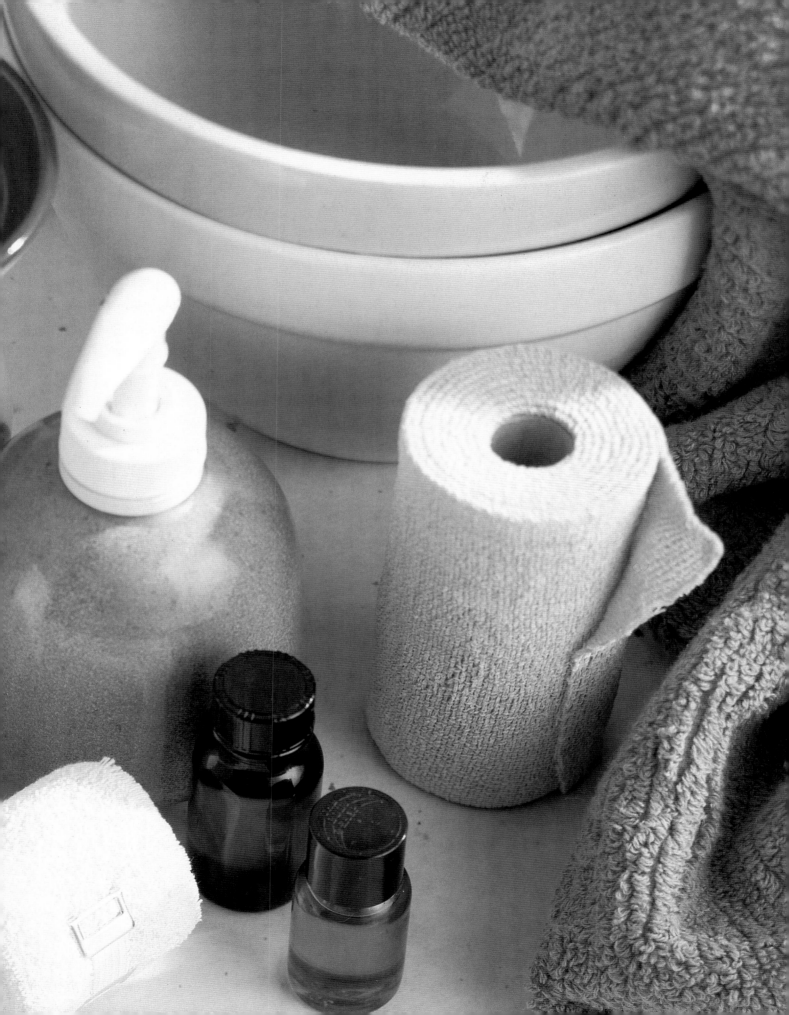

Healing Powers of Essential Oils

While we were living on the herb farm, we used the plants and their oils in skin and hair care products, healing creams and perfumes, as protectives for our pets, ourselves and the gardens, and to enhance the food in our restaurant. Since this time there has scarcely been a day when I have not employed the oils in one way or another. My little heart-shaped box of 'first aid oils' travels with me everywhere and is in constant demand: for a visitor with a headache, a friend who is feeling stressed, or a child with a cut or bruise. There is a panacea for all. Sometimes just the mere sight and smell of the box can effect an improvement!

My aim in this chapter is to share with you a wealth of information about the fascinating and healing world of aromatherapy, and the ways in which the essential oils can improve your health and help to prevent illness. It is empowering and comforting to know that you can easily deal with simple complaints and first aid situations at home

Cautions

The essential oils are toxic and should only be used internally on the advice of a qualified aromatherapist or naturopath.

Keep the essential oils out of the reach of children—they could be lethal if drunk.

Read the cautions associated with any of the oils listed in all the chapters in this book.

Most of the oils should be combined with a carrier oil, such as the sweet almond oil or olive oil, before using on the skin.

Always use the appropriate proportions of the esssential oils and the carrier oil.

Use only the best quality essential oils—there are many synthetic oils available so look for the essential oils that state 'pure' or '100% natural'. The synthetic oils are usually called 'fragrant oil' or 'perfume oil'.

Baths

As discussed in Chapter 1, there are a variety of baths that can be used therapeutically. The warm baths are wonderful for relaxing a stressed mind and body.

Hot baths help to break a dry fever by increasing the pespiration and respiration rates and eliminating any toxins from the body.

Cold baths are used to improve breathing and muscle tone and to decrease fatigue. They also help to improve thyroid function and skin tone and relieve constipation.

Footbaths are an excellent treatment for the beginnings of a cold or 'flu but must be used as soon as any symptoms appear to gain the full benefits. Footbaths also soothe tired, aching feet or sports-worn feet.

There are many other types of baths to enjoy for their therapeutic value, some of these are epsom salts baths, herb baths, milk baths, honey baths and vinegar baths.

Epsom salts baths are made by adding half a box of epsom salts and several drops of your favourite essential oil to a warm bath while the water is running. Soak in the bath for at least twenty minutes to half an hour for aches and pains to melt away.

Herb baths are used for many purposes, mostly for their soothing, hydrating, healing and stimulating actions on the body and skin. Among the many ways to incorporate herbs into the bath, the most common methods are adding a strong infusion or decoction, dried herbs in a little muslin bag added to the bath while it is running and herb oils added to the bath. In all these methods add several drops of essential oils to the bath for increased value.

Milk baths help to make the skin soft and silky. You can add fresh or powdered milk or use buttermilk or yoghurt for a mildly acidic bath. Add the essential oils you choose just before getting into the bath.

Honey baths are an age-old treatment to soften the skin and to treat insomnia. Combine a spoonful of honey with some warm water and a few drops of relaxing essential oils to make a runny mixture then add to the bath and swish well before enjoying it.

Another old remedy for itchy skin is a soothing vinegar bath. Add a cupful of cider vinegar and some drops of soothing essential oils to the bath, swish well then have a good soak.

When preparing a
fomentation, always test the
cloth on the inside of your
wrist before applying
it to a sore area.
Apply the fomentation as
hot as can be comfortably
borne. Cover it to keep the
heat in, and reapply every 2
hours until relief is
obtained.

Compresses, Poultices and Fomentations

A compress is usually a cold application used to reduce inflammation by withdrawing heat from a certain area and so easing swelling and pain, such as that from sprains.

A compress is made by soaking a piece of soft cloth in a bowl of cold water, and then sprinkling it with 10 drops of essential oil. Wring the cloth out to spread the oils evenly; leave enough liquid in the cloth so that it is very moist but does not drip. Apply the cloth to the injured area and replace it when it becomes warm.

A fomentation is a hot application which brings increased blood flow to an area. It eases pain, relaxes spasms, draws pus and relieves congestion.

Fomentations are made in the same way as compresses, but very hot water is used instead of cold.

Healing Ointments

This is a basic recipe for a healing ointment. It makes enough for two 50g (1^2/₃oz) jars. Other essential oils may be substituted.

Basic Healing Ointment

7g (approx ¼oz) beeswax
40g (1¹/₃oz) lanolin
50ml (1¹/₃fl oz) olive, canola or grapeseed oil
1 teaspoon simple tincture of benzoin
20 drops lavender oil
30 drops tea tree oil
5 drops rosemary oil
5 drops thyme oil

Melt the beeswax in a small saucepan, taking care not to overheat. Add the lanolin and mix into wax. Add the olive, canola or grapeseed oil slowly while continuing to stir. Take care not to allow the wax to solidify again, or to overheat the mixture. Remove the saucepan from the heat and allow to cool slightly to just above blood heat.

Combine the tincture and the essential oils and add to mixture, drop by drop. Mix well until no droplets of tincture are visible. Pot up ointment in a dark-coloured glass jar when it begins to thicken.

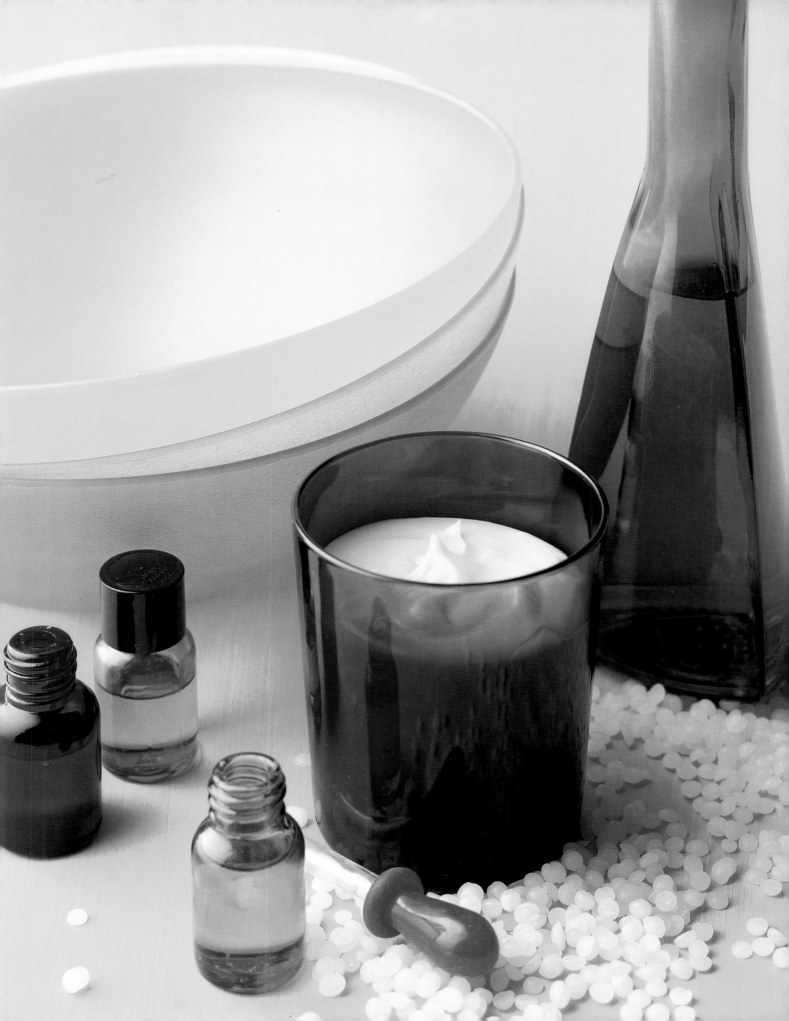

Gargles

Gargles are used to help to relieve hoarseness and voice loss, to ease pain, or to help avoid or reduce infection in the throat.

Add 1 drop of essential oil to 1 cup (250ml/8fl oz) of warm water. Gargle and spit; do not swallow.

Inhalations

Inhalations are used to relieve chest, nasal or sinus congestion, to loosen mucus, and to ease headaches and sore throats.

To make an inhalation, have a towel and a bowl of boiling water ready. Quickly add up to 6 drops of essential oil (depending on your age, or the age of the person) to the bowl, pull the towel over your head and the bowl and inhale the aromatic steam. Always be careful to place the bowl on a non-slip surface. If the patient is very young, very old or frail, the inhalation should take place in the bathroom where the bowl of boiling water may be put in the washbasin for safety, and the patient seated near to the steam.

Stay indoors for some time after an inhalation to prevent damage to mucous membranes made sensitive by the hot steam.

If using thyme or peppermint oil in an inhalation, never use more than 1 to 2 drops.

Lotions

A lotion may be used to wash the face if the skin is very sensitive or troubled with acne, spots or other skin problems. It may also be used as a moisturiser with the addition of 1 teaspoonful of almond oil, or other fine-textured oil.

Skin Lotion

50ml (1^2/3fl oz) rosewater
50ml (1^2/3fl oz) purified water, less 1 teaspoon
1/4–1/2 teaspoon glycerine (try 1/4 first, and increase if liked)
10 drops essential oil

Mix all the ingredients together in a 100ml (3^1/3fl oz) bottle. Shake well to blend thoroughly. Leave for 4 days, shaking occasionally. Filter lotion through coffee filter paper. Store in a dark-coloured glass bottle. Shake before use.

Massage Creams

This recipe is for a simple but very effective massage cream. The essential oils may be chosen according to the complaint being treated—for instance, juniper, pine and rosemary could be the choice if rheumatism is being treated.

This cream should not be refrigerated. The thickness may be adjusted to your own preference by using more or less olive or canola oil.

Massage Cream

30ml (1fl oz) olive or canola oil
125g (4oz) Copha (hydrogenated coconut cooking fat)
5 drops simple tincture of benzoin
60 drops essential oil

Melt the oil and Copha together in a saucepan over a gentle heat. Remove from heat and allow to cool slightly. Mix together the tincture and the essential oil. Add this to the cream mixture and beat well, continuing to beat until cold. Pot up cream in dark-coloured glass jars.

Massage Oils

This is a basic massage oil blend. The essential oils may be chosen according to the complaint being treated—for instance, lavender, black pepper and rosemary could be chosen if muscular and joint stiffness is being treated.

It is a good idea to make up 100ml ($3^1/_3$fl oz) of the massage oil base, excluding the essential oils. This base can then be divided into four 25ml (approx. 1fl oz) bottles and essential oils for different purposes may be added to each one. If you choose this system, be sure to divide the essential oil content in the following recipe by 4 to 10 drops to each 25ml approx. 1fl oz) bottle.

Basic Massage Oil

70ml (2$^1/_3$fl oz) grapeseed or canola oil
2 teaspoons almond oil
2 teaspoons avocado oil
1 teaspoon wheat germ oil (this helps to prevent rancidity)
20–40 drops essential oil

Mouthwashes

A mouthwash is used to help sweeten the breath, and to heal sores, ulcers and gum problems.

Mouthwashes are made by adding 4 drops of essential oil to 25ml (approx. 1fl oz) of brandy. Add 1 teaspoon of the mouthwash mixture to $\frac{1}{4}$ cup (60ml/2fl oz) of warm water. Rinse mouth, but do not swallow the mixture.

Oil burners

Oil burners are a lovely way in which to fill the air with a pleasant aroma. The perfume is gentle yet pervasive. Usually two ceramic dishes are arranged one on top of the other. The bottom container has air holes and a candle is placed inside it. The top part holds water into which a few drops of essential oil are sprinkled. Suitable candles are those which are used in food warmers or night lights; they burn for about five hours and are smokeless. The deeper the top container is, the better, as it is not good to let the water evaporate completely.

Wound Wash

Wound washes are used to cleanse wounds which are contaminated with dirt.

They are made by adding 5 to 10 drops (depending on the age of the patient) of essential oil(s) to 100ml ($3\frac{1}{3}$fl oz) of warm or cold boiled water. The water should be agitated before being used to avoid the possibility of 'hot spots' of oil.

Oil burners and scented candles made with pure essential oils diffuse the oils gradually into a room

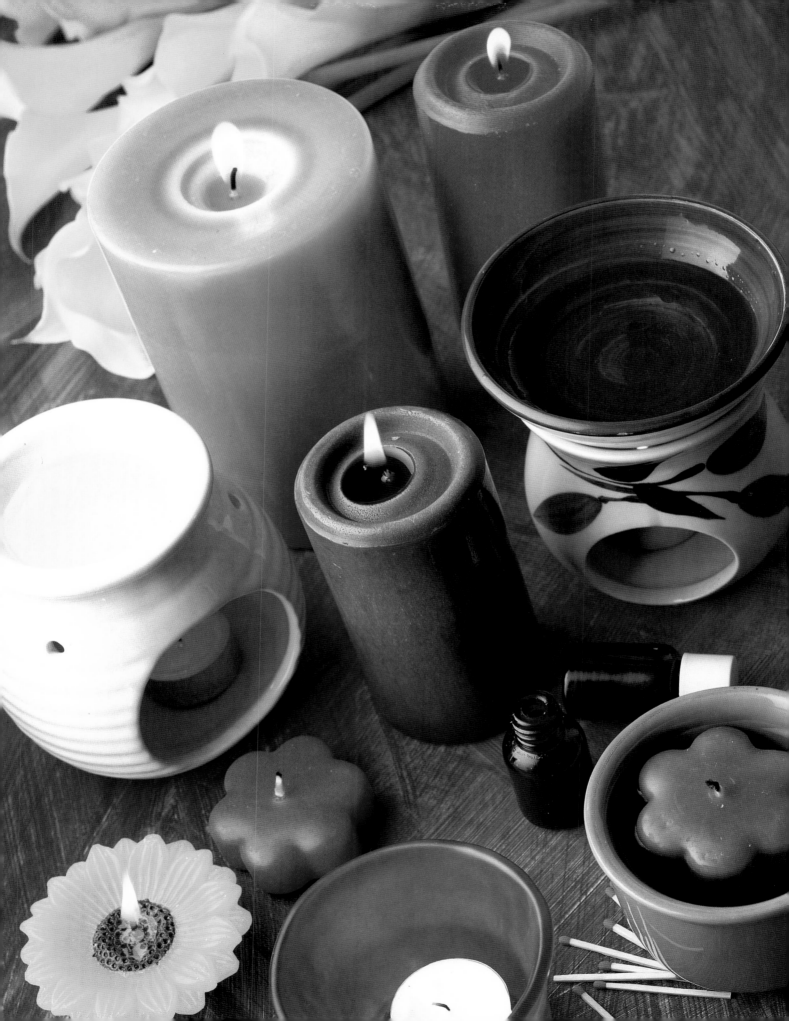

First Aid Box

Every home and car should have a well-equipped first aid box. The ability to give prompt assistance can often prevent excessive pain and trauma and, in some cases, save a life. The following first aid box contents are in addition to the usual bandages, sticking plasters and scissors, and are used to mix the essential oils, according to the remedy instructions.

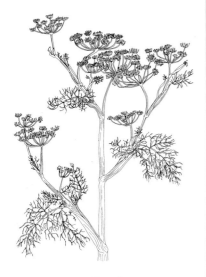

Fennel

2 empty dropper bottles
2 eye-droppers
15ml ($\frac{1}{2}$fl oz) bottle almond oil
15ml ($\frac{1}{2}$fl oz) bottle brandy
50ml ($1\frac{2}{3}$fl oz) witch hazel extract
50ml ($1\frac{2}{3}$fl oz) purified water
Basic Healing Ointment (see page 64)

Essential oils to include
(the most important ones are marked with *):

Benzoin	Fennel	Mint
Bergamot	*Geranium	Myrrh
Black Pepper	Ginger	*Peppermint
Cedarwood	Hyssop	Pine
*Chamomile,	Juniper	Rosemary
German or Roman	*Lavender	*Spearmint
Clary Sage	*Lemon	*Tea Tree
Cypress	Marjoram	*Thyme
*Eucalyptus		

The Essential Oils for Healing

Most essential oils have healing properties, but some are more efficacious than others. The following list contains descriptions of twenty-three oils used in this section for health and healing. The most useful first aid oils are marked with an asterisk (*). These oils are the best ones with which to start your 'oil pharmacy'; they also have the advantage of being (with a couple of exceptions) the least expensive oils.

The properties listed for each oil are only those applicable to healing.

If you can only afford a couple of oils to begin with, I would urge you to make lavender and tea tree your first purchases, followed closely by chamomile and geranium. After you read through the remedies, you will notice immediately how often these remarkable oils are used. Lavender, in particular, has the advantage also of being gentle and safe enough to use for the whole family, ranging from a new baby only two days old to a frail great-grandmother who is ninety-two years of age!

I have avoided including the three oils which are among the most expensive, namely rose, neroli and jasmine. There are other less expensive oils which are very suitable for medicinal purposes and which are far less costly.

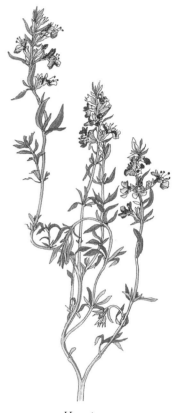

Hyssop

Cautions

Some of the essential oils are very toxic and should only be used internally on the advice of a qualified aromatherapist or naturopath.

Many of the oils are unsuitable to use if certain conditions exist, such as epilepsy or pregnancy. Please note the cautions at the end of each relevant entry.

Benzoin

Styrax benzoin

USE FOR: Antiseptic, anti-inflammatory, antioxidant, mild stimulant. Arthritis, gout, poor circulation, rheumatism. Cystitis, vaginal discharges. Asthma, bronchitis, coughs, chills, colds, laryngitis. Fungal infections of the skin, skin irritations.

Bergamot

Citrus bergamia

USE FOR: Antiseptic, acne, cold sores, eczema, psoriasis, scabies, thrush, pruritus. Cystitis, other urinary infections. Varicose ulcers. Mouth infections, sore throat, tonsillitis. Colds, fever, influenza, infectious diseases. Anxiety, depression, stress-related disorders. CAUTION: This oil can cause irritation if used on sensitive skin. It is also phototoxic—do not use on exposed skin during long exposure to sunlight or pigmentation may occur.

Black Pepper

Piper nigrum

USE FOR: Analgesic, antiseptic, pain-relieving, fever-reducing. Chilblains. Anaemia. Arthritis, rheumatism, muscular aches and pains, sprains, strains, muscular stiffness, neuralgia, poor circulation. Catarrh, chills, influenza, other viral infections. Colic, constipation, diarrhoea, flatulence, nausea.

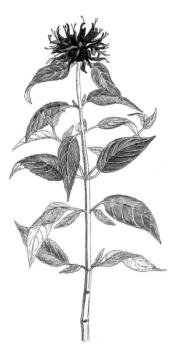

Bergamot

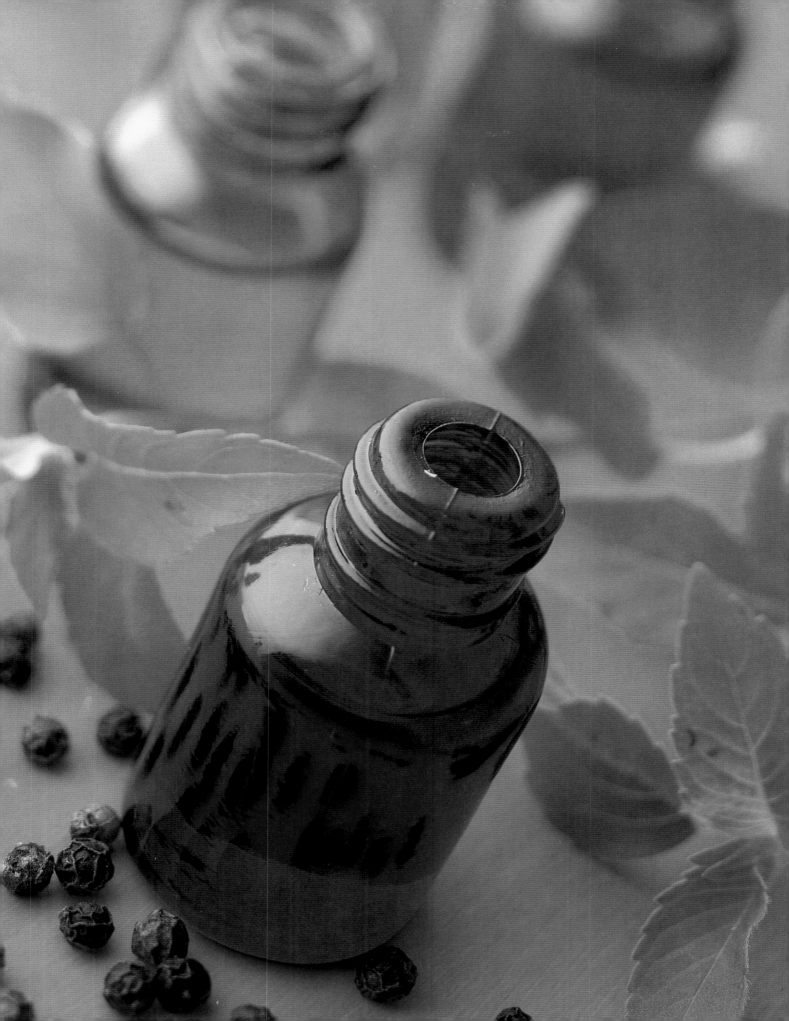

Cedarwood

Juniperus virginiana; Cedrus atlantica

USE FOR: Antiseptic, arthritis, rheumatism. Acne, eczema, dermatitis, fungal infections. Urinary tract problems. Leucorrhoea, thrush. Bronchitis, coughs, catarrh. Nervous tension, stress-related problems.

CAUTION: Not to be used internally. Not to be used during pregnancy. An irritant to some sensitive skins.

*Chamomile, German or Roman

Anthemis nobilis; Matricaria chamomilla

USE FOR: Acne, dermatitis, allergies, arthritis, inflamed joints, rheumatism. Boils, burns, cuts. Flatulence, diarrhoea. Headaches, insomnia, nervous tension. Inflammation, insect bites, rashes. Sprains, strains, wounds. Menopausal problems. Babies teething pain and colic.

CAUTION: A skin irritant to some people.

Clary Sage

Salvia sclarea

USE FOR: Acne, boils, dandruff, hair loss. High blood pressure, muscular aches and pains. Asthma, throat infections, whooping cough. Labour pain, period pain, Leucorrhoea. Depression, impotence, nervous tension. Colic, cramp, flatulence.

CAUTION: Inhalation or other use of large doses of this oil can cause severe headache and poisoning. Not to be used during pregnancy.

Cypress

Cupressus sempervirens

USE FOR: Circulatory stimulant, menopausal problems. Cold hands and feet. Haemorrhoids, varicose veins, pyorrhoea. Coughs, laryngitis, colds. Muscle cramps, rheumatism. Oedema. Menopausal problems. Nervous tension.

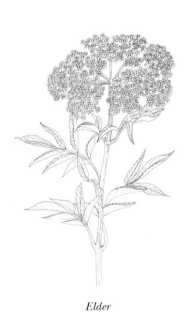

Elder

*Eucalyptus

Eucalyptus globulus and other species

USE FOR: Burns, antiseptic, blisters, cuts, herpes, head lice, insect bites, insect repellent, wounds. Muscular aches and pains, rheumatoid arthritis. Asthma, bronchitis, catarrh, coughs, sinusitis, throat infections. Cystitis, leucorrhoea. Chickenpox, measles, influenza.

Fennel

Foeniculum vulgare

USE FOR: Liver cleanser. Digestive. Colic, constipation, indigestion, flatulence, nausea. Menopausal irregularities. Obesity (affects hormones), cellulite, fluid retention. Bruises, pyorrhoea. Asthma, bronchitis.

CAUTION: Phototoxic. Not to be used on skin before exposure to sunlight. Not to be used internally, during pregnancy or by people with epilepsy.

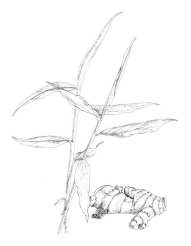

Ginger

*Geranium

Pelargonium odoratissima and other species

USE FOR: Acne, bruises, burns, scalds (minor), dermatitis, eczema, head lice, ringworm. Engorged breasts, menopausal problems, premenstrual syndrome (PMS). Poor circulation. Sore throat, tonsillitis. Wounds. Nervous tension, neuralgia.

Ginger

Zingiber officinale

USE FOR: Arthritis, rheumatism, muscular aches and pains, poor circulation, sprains, strains. Catarrh, coughs, sore throat. Stomach cramps, nausea, travel sickness. Chills, colds, influenza, fever. Nervous exhaustion.

Hyssop
Hyssopus officinalis
MEDICINAL PROPERTIES: Raises and lowers blood pressure. Expectorant. Digestive. Cardiovascular tonic.

USE FOR: Asthma, coughs, emphysema, catarrh. Flatulence, colic, mild constipation, gastroenteritis. Leucorrhoea. Bruises, dermatitis, eczema, inflammation, wounds. Fatigue, nervous tension.

CAUTION: Toxic in large doses. Never to be used by epileptics or during pregnancy.

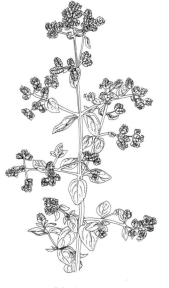

Marjoram

Juniper
Juniperus communis
USE FOR: Purifying air in sick rooms. Relief of urine retention. Haemorrhoids (well diluted). Removes toxins, gout. Colds, influenza, infectious diseases. Most period problems. Acne, dermatitis, eczema. Muscular pain. Anxiety, nervous tension.

CAUTION: Not to be used during pregnancy.

*Lavender
Lavandula angustifolia
USE FOR: Abscesses, acne, allergies, athlete's foot, asthma, bruises, burns, sunburn and scalds (minor), sores, spots, dermatitis, eczema, inflammations, insect bites and stings, boils, scabies, ringworm. Bad breath, bronchitis, catarrh, laryngitis, throat infections. Insect repellent. Cystitis. Depression, headaches, nausea, insomnia, nervous tension. Lumbago, muscular aches and pains, rheumatism. Wounds.

*Lemon
Citrus limonum
USE FOR: Digestive. Circulatory stimulant. Acne, boils, chilblains, corns, cuts, insect bites, mouth ulcers, spots, warts. Asthma, bronchitis, catarrh, colds and influenza, throat infections, fevers. Arthritis and rheumatism, poor circulation, varicose veins. High blood pressure. Indigestion.

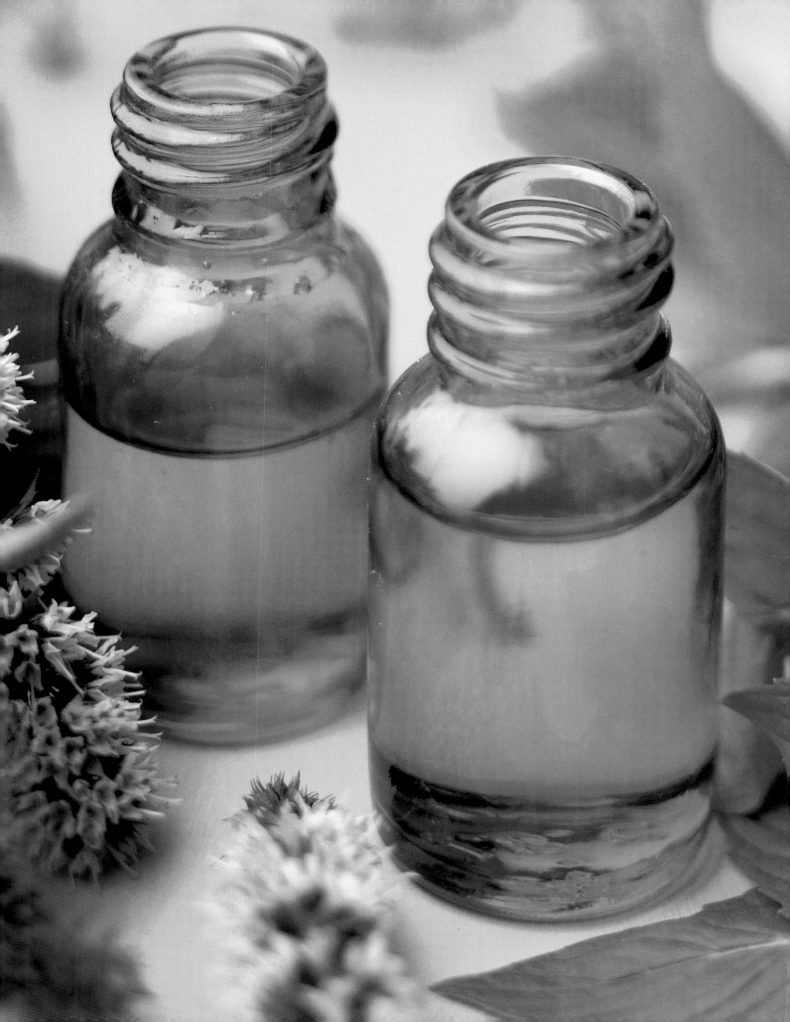

Marjoram

Origanum majorana

USE FOR: Analgesic. Arthritis, chilblains, lumbago, sprains, bruises, rheumatism, joint and muscle pain. Asthma, bronchitis, coughs, colds. Colic, indigestion, constipation. Headache, migraine, premenstrual syndrome (PMS) and fainting.

CAUTION: Not to be used during pregnancy.

Mint

See Peppermint and Spearmint

Myrrh

Commiphora myrrha

USE FOR: Arthritis. Asthma, bronchitis, catarrh, coughs, colds. Athlete's foot, eczema, ringworm, wounds. Gum infections, mouth ulcers, gingivitis, sore throat. Thrush, leucorrhoea, pruritus. Diarrhoea, indigestion, flatulence. Haemorrhoids.

CAUTION: Not to be used during pregnancy.

*Peppermint

Mentha piperita

USE FOR: Acne, dermatitis, ringworm, scabies. Asthma, bronchitis, colds, influenza and fever. Colic, indigestion, nausea. Fainting, headache, mental fatigue, nervous stress, palpitations. Bad breath. Muscular pain, neuralgia.

CAUTION: Use in smaller quantities than for other oils —1% is plenty. Never use during pregnancy.

Pine

Pinus sylvestris

USE FOR: Arthritis, rheumatism, muscular aches and pains, poor circulation. Scabies, cuts, head lice. Asthma, bronchitis, catarrh, coughs, sinusitis, sores, sore throat, colds, influenza. Cystitis, urinary infections. Fatigue, nervous exhaustion.

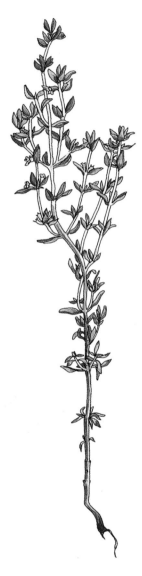

Common Thyme

Rosemary

Rosmarinus officinalis

USE FOR: Acne, dermatitis, eczema, scabies. Arteriosclerosis.
Asthma, bronchitis, colds, influenza, fevers. Colitis, flatulence,
fluid retention. Headaches, hypotension. Infections. Leucorrhoea.
Liver problems. Nervous exhaustion, palpitations. Poor
circulation, rheumatism, muscular pain, gout. Varicose veins.
Whooping cough.
CAUTION: Not to be used during pregnancy or by people with
epilepsy.

*Spearmint

Mentha spicata

USE FOR: The properties and uses of spearmint are similar to those
of peppermint but are less powerful, making the oil more suitable
for children and during pregnancy.

*Tea tree

Melaleuca alternifolia

USE FOR: Abscesses, acne, asthma, athlete's foot, blisters, boils,
burns and scalds (minor), warts, wounds. Bronchitis, catarrh,
colds, influenza, fevers, coughs, sinusitis. Infectious diseases. Insect
bites. Nappy rash. Cystitis, thrush, vaginitis. Tuberculosis,
whooping cough.

*Thyme

Thymus vulgaris, T. citriodorus and chemotype linalol

T. citriodorus and chemotype linalol are the safest to use for
children as they are far less toxic than T. vulgaris.
USE FOR: Abscesses, acne, bruises, burns and scalds (minor),
dermatitis, eczema, insect bites. Arthritis, rheumatism. Asthma,
bronchitis, catarrh, chills, colds, fevers, coughs, croup. Cystitis.
Headaches. Infectious diseases. Insomnia, nervous debility, stress.
CAUTION: A very powerful oil. Use only $\frac{1}{2}$–1%. Never use neat. Never
use during pregnancy.

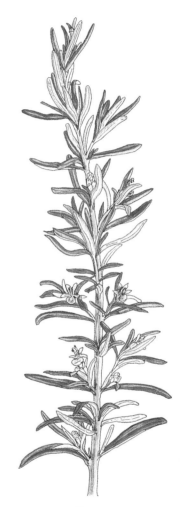

Rosemary

Remedies

Many of these remedies should be used either as first aid procedures or in conjunction with professional treatment. Home treatment of long-standing or serious complaints is neither safe nor advisable.

Methods for making and using these treatments will be found earlier in this chapter.

Abrasions

ESSENTIAL OILS
Tea tree, lavender

TREATMENT
Wound wash using single or mixed oils. Repeat every 2 hours if necessary. Leave uncovered if possible. If a sticking plaster is needed, use 1 drop of either of the oils on the plaster pad, or apply Healing Ointment.

Abscesses

ESSENTIAL OILS
Chamomile, lavender, tea tree

TREATMENT
Fomentation of all the oils. Apply 2 hourly.

Anaemia

ESSENTIAL OILS
Black pepper, lemon, peppermint

TREATMENT
Use singly or in combination for baths and massage.

Anal Fistula (Abscess)

ESSENTIAL OILS

Lavender, tea tree, geranium

TREATMENT

Bathe the area with warm water to which you have added 5 drops of tea tree oil. Make a Massage Cream containing the above oils. Massage the cream around the anal area twice daily.

Arteriosclerosis

ESSENTIAL OILS

Juniper, black pepper, rosemary

TREATMENT

Massage. Bath.

Arthritis—Osteoarthritis

ESSENTIAL OILS

Cedarwood, black pepper, rosemary

TREATMENT

Use singly or, for much better results, in combination for massage and baths.

Arthritis—Rheumatoid

ESSENTIAL OILS

Rosemary, juniper, ginger

TREATMENT

Use singly or, for much better results, in combination for massage and baths.

Asthma, Children

ESSENTIAL OILS

Lavender, geranium

TREATMENT

Bath. Massage.

Asthma, Adult

ESSENTIAL OILS

Tea tree, lavender, clary sage

TREATMENT

Bath. Massage.

Athlete's Foot

ESSENTIAL OILS

Tea tree, myrrh, thyme

TREATMENT

For a footbath, use 1 drop of each oil in a bowl (big enough for both feet) containing warm water. Add 2 drops of each oil to 1 teaspoon of vegetable oil. Massage the whole foot and between the toes, 4 times a day if possible. Add 2 drops of each oil to 1 cup (150g/5oz) of unperfumed talcum powder. Dust the feet before wearing shoes and socks. Pre-soak socks in water containing 10 drops of tea tree oil and wash separately from the family wash.

Bee Stings

ESSENTIAL OILS

Chamomile, lavender

TREATMENT

Scrape the sting out sideways; do not pull it out. Mix 1 drop of each oil with 1 teaspoon of bicarbonate of soda (this counteracts the acidity of the sting) and enough water to make a soft paste. Apply to the painful area. Repeat hourly, or more often if needed.

Black Eye

ESSENTIAL OILS

Lavender, chamomile

TREATMENT

Compress using 1 drop of each oil mixed well into a mixture of 1 tablespoon of ice-cold witch hazel and 2 teaspoons of ice-cold water. Use the compress over the entire eye area, keeping the eye closed during treatment.

Bleeding, External

ESSENTIAL OILS

Geranium, lemon, cypress

TREATMENT

Apply a cold compress (witch hazel, if possible) containing the above oils. Bandage firmly, but not too tightly, in place.

Blisters

ESSENTIAL OILS

Lavender, tea tree

TREATMENT

Apply 2 drops of either of the above oils, neat. Massage in gently. Do not break the blister.

Boils and Carbuncles

ESSENTIAL OILS

Bergamot, lavender, tea tree

TREATMENT

Wash the affected area and surrounding skin 3 times daily with
2 drops of bergamot and 2 drops of lavender oil mixed in 50ml
(1²⁄₃fl oz) of warm, boiled water. Smooth on a mixture of 5 drops
of tea tree oil in 1 teaspoon of vegetable oil.

Breath Sweetener

ESSENTIAL OILS

Bergamot, peppermint, myrrh

TREATMENT

Make a Mouthwash using the above essential oils and use as often
as needed.

Bronchitis

ESSENTIAL OILS

Benzoin, marjoram, eucalyptus

TREATMENT

Inhalation and chest massage, using a blend of the oils.

Bruises

ESSENTIAL OILS

Geranium, chamomile, rosemary

TREATMENT

Hold a bag of frozen peas or ice blocks wrapped in cloth on the
area for a few minutes. Massage with a blend of 6 drops of the
above essential oils in 1 tablespoon of vegetable oil.

Burns, Minor

ESSENTIAL OILS

Lavender

TREATMENT

Hold the burn under cold water or use ice water compresses for
10 full minutes. Gently pat on neat lavender oil. Cover with a dry
dressing.

Cold Sores

ESSENTIAL OILS

Tea tree, lavender

TREATMENT

Apply either oil neat to sore.

Constipation

ESSENTIAL OILS

Black pepper, rosemary

TREATMENT

Make a Massage Oil containing the above essential oils. Massage
the abdomen daily in a clockwise direction.

Coughs and Colds

ESSENTIAL OILS

Eucalyptus, thyme, lemon, rosemary

TREATMENT

Use the above essential oils in the bath, massage and inhalation.

Conjunctivitis

ESSENTIAL OILS

Chamomile, lemon

TREATMENT

Compress using 1 drop of each oil mixed well into a mixture of 1 tablespoon of ice-cold witch hazel and 2 teaspoons of ice-cold water. Use the compress over the entire eye area, keeping the eye closed during treatment.

Catarrh

ESSENTIAL OILS

Peppermint, tea tree, rosemary

TREATMENT

Inhalation. Massage on chest and back. Oil burner.

Chickenpox

ESSENTIAL OILS

Lavender

TREATMENT

Add 10 drops of essential oil (a drop at a time to prevent lumping) to 1 cup (180g/6oz) of bicarbonate of soda. Mix 1 or 2 teaspoons with enough cold water to make a milky lotion. Use cottonwool balls to dab the lotion onto the itchy spots. Repeat as often as needed. Add bicarbonate of soda and 4 drops of lavender oil to a warm bath to soothe the itching, and to calm the patient.

Chilblains

ESSENTIAL OILS

Lemon, lavender, rosemary

TREATMENT

Massage initially with neat lavender oil. Make a blend of the above oils with vegetable oil and use to massage area daily.

Cradle Cap

ESSENTIAL OILS

Chamomile, lavender

TREATMENT

Make a Massage Oil using 5 drops of chamomile oil and 8 drops of
lavender oil in 80ml (2⅔fl oz) of sweet almond oil and
1 tablespoon of olive oil. This oil may also be used as a general
massage oil for babies.

Cramps, Muscular

ESSENTIAL OILS

Lavender, black pepper, rosemary

TREATMENT

Blend the above essential oils with vegetable oil for massage. Use
3 drops of each oil in a bath.

Cuts

ESSENTIAL OILS

Lavender, tea tree

TREATMENT

Compress to stop bleeding. Leave open to the air unless severe. If
necessary, put 2 drops of either oil on a dressing to cover.

Cystic Breast Disease

ESSENTIAL OILS

Lavender, chamomile, geranium

TREATMENT

Massage, using 3% total essential oils.

Cystitis

ESSENTIAL OILS

Bergamot, benzoin, cedarwood

TREATMENT

1 drop each of bergamot and benzoin plus 2 drops of cedarwood
in 2 teaspoons of vegetable oil to massage over bladder area. Add
3 drops of each to a hot bath.

Debility, Physical

ESSENTIAL OILS

Peppermint, rosemary, geranium

TREATMENT

Baths. Massage. Inhalation. Air spray. Oil burner.

Dermatitis

ESSENTIAL OILS

Chamomile, lavender, cedarwood

TREATMENT

Add 3 drops of each essential oil to a bath. Mix 2 drops of each in
2 teaspoons of vegetable oil to be used as a topical application.
Mix 4 drops of lavender oil in 2 teaspoons of cider vinegar and
apply topically to ease itching.

Diarrhoea

ESSENTIAL OILS

Peppermint

TREATMENT

Mix 1 drop with 1 teaspoon of honey in a glass of warm water
and sip slowly.

Dog Bite

ESSENTIAL OILS

Thyme, lavender, tea tree

TREATMENT

Wash the area immediately with Wound Wash using the above
essential oils. Apply neat tea tree oil to the wound and cover with a
light dressing. Go straight to hospital if the skin is broken as you
may need a tetanus injection.

Earache

ESSENTIAL OILS

Tea tree

TREATMENT

Mix 3 drops of tea tree oil in 1 teaspoon of olive oil which has been warmed to blood heat (no hotter). Drip a few drops in the ear. Plug the external opening of the ear with cottonwool. If earache is persistent or severe, seek professional help.

Eczema

ESSENTIAL OILS

Bergamot, lavender, chamomile

TREATMENT

Add 3 drops of each essential oil to a bath. Mix 2 drops of each in 2 teaspoons of vegetable oil to be used as a topical application. Mix 4 drops of lavender oil in 2 teaspoons of cider vinegar and apply topically to ease itching.

Endometriosis

ESSENTIAL OILS

Geranium, clary sage, cypress

TREATMENT

Massage lower abdomen using a blend containing 3% of these essential oils. Sitz bath, using 4 drops of each oil.

Exhaustion, Physical

ESSENTIAL OILS

Lavender, peppermint, geranium

TREATMENT

Bath. Massage. Inhale scent of blended oils. Oil burner.

Exhaustion, Nervous

ESSENTIAL OILS
Chamomile, peppermint, clary sage
TREATMENT
Bath. Massage. Inhale scent of blended oils. Oil burner.

Fainting

ESSENTIAL OILS
Marjoram, lavender
TREATMENT
Put a few drops of essential oil(s) on a paper tissue and hold it under the nose of the faint person; or, sniff directly from the bottle. Oil burner. Smelling salts.

Smelling Salts

20 drops marjoram oil
10 drops peppermint oil
20 drops lavender oil
4 tablespoons coarse sea salt crystals

Mix the oils together and sprinkle over the sea salt crystals. Pack mixture into a small jar and seal tightly. Sniff the contents to restore equilibrium if feeling faint, or when a tension headache is a problem.

Fatigue

ESSENTIAL OILS
Lemon, clary sage, lavender
TREATMENT
Bath. Massage. Inhale scent of blended oils. Oil burner.

Fever

ESSENTIAL OILS
Black pepper, lavender, peppermint
TREATMENT
Hot bath. Massage.

Fibrositis

ESSENTIAL OILS

Black pepper, peppermint, rosemary

TREATMENT

Massage. Bath.

Flu

ESSENTIAL OILS

Tea tree, peppermint, black pepper

TREATMENT

Hot bath. Massage.

Frozen Shoulder

ESSENTIAL OILS

Rosemary, black pepper, chamomile

TREATMENT

Massage.

German Measles

ESSENTIAL OILS

Lavender

TREATMENT

Add 10 drops of essential oil (a drop at a time to prevent lumping) to 1 cup (180g/6oz) of bicarbonate of soda. Mix 1 or 2 teaspoons with enough cold water to make a milky lotion. Use cottonwool balls to dab the lotion onto the itchy spots. Repeat as often as needed. Add bicarbonate of soda and 4 drops of lavender oil to a warm bath to soothe the itching, and to calm the patient.

Glandular Fever

ESSENTIAL OILS

Cypress, tea tree, lemon

TREATMENT

Bath. Gently massage swollen glands using 2 drops of each
essential oil in 2 teaspoons of vegetable oil.

Gum Infections

ESSENTIAL OILS

Tea tree, myrrh

TREATMENT

Mouthwash, using either or both essential oils.

Haemorrhoids

ESSENTIAL OILS

Cypress, juniper, geranium

TREATMENT

Add 2 drops of each essential oil to half a bowlful (large enough to
sit in) of warm water. Agitate the water to disperse the oils. Sit in
the water for 10 to 15 minutes. Follow by gently massaging the
haemorrhoids with 1 drop of each oil in 1 tablespoon of olive oil.

Hayfever

ESSENTIAL OILS

Lavender, lemon, geranium, hyssop

TREATMENT

Inhalation. Bath. Oil burner.

Headaches and Migraine, Nervous

ESSENTIAL OILS

Lavender, marjoram

TREATMENT

Hot and cold footbath. Bath. Inhalation, using 2 drops of either
essential oil in 2 tablespoons of hot cider vinegar. Neck massage.
Oil burner. Smelling bottle.

Smelling Bottle

45ml (1½fl oz) cider vinegar
30 drops lavender oil
20 drops rosemary oil
15 drops peppermint oil
15 drops marjoram oil

Mix all ingredients in a 100ml (3⅓fl oz) dark-coloured glass
bottle. Shake well. Leave for 1 week, shaking daily. Strain mixture
through coffee filter paper. Add 50ml (2fl oz) of purified water.
Store in a cool, dark place. Decant some of the mixture into a
small bottle and carry it with you; inhale to ease headaches, clear
the brain and lessen tension.

Headaches and Migraine, Gastric

ESSENTIAL OILS

Peppermint

TREATMENT

Make a Massage Oil and massage over stomach and abdomen.
Inhalation. Bath.

Head Lice

ESSENTIAL OILS

Rosemary, lavender, eucalyptus

TREATMENT

Add 5 drops of each essential oil to 1 tablespoon of olive oil. Massage mixture into the hair, paying particular attention to the area behind the ears. Cover the head with a shower cap and leave on overnight. Wash the hair in the morning, using 2 drops of rosemary oil in the final rinse. When hair is dry, comb it with a fine-toothed comb (available from pharmacies). Repeat the treatment a week later, but do not continue on a regular basis.

Heartburn

ESSENTIAL OILS

Peppermint

TREATMENT

Mix 1 drop with 1 teaspoon of honey in a glass of lukewarm water and sip slowly.

Hives

ESSENTIAL OILS

Bergamot, lavender, chamomile

TREATMENT

Add 3 drops of each essential oil to a bath. Mix 2 drops of each in 2 teaspoons of vegetable oil to be used as a topical application. Mix 4 drops of lavender oil in 2 teaspoons of cider vinegar and apply topically to ease itching.

Hoarseness and Voice Loss

ESSENTIAL OILS

Lavender, myrrh, thyme

TREATMENT

Gargle. Inhalation. Massage of throat.

Hypertension
ESSENTIAL OILS
Marjoram, hyssop, lavender
TREATMENT
Bath. Massage. Air spray. Oil burner.

Immune System Booster
ESSENTIAL OILS
Tea tree, eucalyptus, thyme
TREATMENT
Bath. Massage. Air spray. Oil burner.

Indigestion
ESSENTIAL OIL
Peppermint, ginger
TREATMENT
Mix 1 drop of either essential oil with 1 teaspoon of honey and place in a glass. Fill glass with lukewarm water, mixing contents well. Sip slowly.

Inflammation
ESSENTIAL OILS
Chamomile, lavender, hyssop
TREATMENT
Cold Compress.

Insomnia, Children

ESSENTIAL OILS
Chamomile, lavender
TREATMENT
Warm bath. Massage. Inhalation.

Insomnia, Adults

ESSENTIAL OILS
Chamomile, lavender, marjoram
TREATMENT
Bath. Massage. Air spray. Oil burner.

'Jock Itch'

ESSENTIAL OILS
Tea tree, lavender
TREATMENT
Add 5 drops of each essential oil to 1 tablespoon of olive oil.
Massage into itchy area after carefully washing and drying
the groin area.

Laryngitis

ESSENTIAL OILS
Benzoin, thyme, lavender
TREATMENT
Gargle. Throat massage. Inhalation.

Lumbago

ESSENTIAL OILS
Ginger, rosemary, marjoram
TREATMENT
Bath. Massage.

M.E. (Myalgic Encephalomyelitis or 'Yuppie flu')

ESSENTIAL OILS

Grapefruit, cypress, rosemary

TREATMENT

Massage. Bath. Air spray. Oil burner.

Measles

ESSENTIAL OILS

Lavender, eucalyptus

TREATMENT

Use the lavender essential oil in the same way as for Chickenpox. Complete bed-rest is essential for patients with measles, as complications can occur. Use eucalyptus and lavender oils in an Air Spray through the whole house to help prevent the spread of the disease.

Menopause, Hot Flushes

ESSENTIAL OILS

Clary sage, geranium, lemon

TREATMENT

Bath. Massage. Air spray. Oil burner.

Menopause, Depression

ESSENTIAL OILS

Lavender, clary sage, bergamot

TREATMENT

Bath. Massage. Air spray. Oil burner.

Menstrual Cramps

ESSENTIAL OILS

Bergamot, clary sage, cypress

TREATMENT

Bath. Massage. Air spray. Oil burner.

Menstruation, Heavy Loss

ESSENTIAL OILS

Geranium, lemon, chamomile

TREATMENT

Bath. Massage. Air spray. Oil burner.

Menstruation, Irregular

ESSENTIAL OILS

Clary sage, geranium, chamomile

TREATMENT

Bath. Massage. Air spray. Oil burner.

Menstruation, Painful

ESSENTIAL OILS

Juniper, clary sage, marjoram

TREATMENT

Bath. Massage. Air spray. Oil burner.

Menstruation, Scanty

ESSENTIAL OILS

Myrrh, marjoram, clary sage

TREATMENT

Bath. Massage. Air spray. Oil burner.

Morning Sickness

ESSENTIAL OILS

Spearmint, lavender

TREATMENT

Place 2 drops of spearmint oil on cottonwool, and tuck it under your pillow. Place 1 drop of spearmint oil and 2 drops of lavender oil in a bowl of warm water placed close to the bed before retiring.

Mosquito, Gnat and Fly Bites and Stings

ESSENTIAL OILS
Lavender

TREATMENT
Apply neat oil until pain is relieved.

Mouth Ulcers

ESSENTIAL OILS
Myrrh, clary sage

TREATMENT
Mouthwash.

Mucus

ESSENTIAL OILS
Benzoin, black pepper, tea tree

TREATMENT
Inhalation. Bath. Chest massage.

Mumps

ESSENTIAL OILS
Lavender, tea tree, lemon

TREATMENT
Bed rest. Gently massage sore, swollen glands and the whole neck area with a blend of 2 drops of lavender oil, 1 drop of tea tree oil and 2 drops of lemon oil in 1 tablespoon of olive oil.

Muscular Aches and Pains

ESSENTIAL OILS
Black pepper, marjoram, rosemary

TREATMENT
Use a mixture of the oils in Massage and Baths.

Nappy Rash

ESSENTIAL OILS
Lavender, chamomile, tea tree
TREATMENT
Wash baby's bottom, using cottonwool and warm water to which
you have added 2 drops of tea tree oil for every 500ml (16fl oz) of
warm water. Agitate the water well before using. Dry skin gently
and use either Nappy Rash Powder or Healing Ointment ,
containing the above essential oils.

Nappy Rash Powder

1 cup (155g/5oz) cornflour
1 tablespoon zinc oxide powder (available from pharmacies)
5 drops lavender oil
5 drops tea tree oil

Mix the cornflour and zinc oxide powder together very well. Mix
the essential oils together and add to powder, 1 drop at a time. Stir
constantly, or the powder will form lumps. Allow the powder to
stand for 4 days to blend completely, shaking or stirring
occasionally to mix. Store in an airtight container.

Nausea and Vomiting

ESSENTIAL OIL
Peppermint, lavender
TREATMENT
Mix 1 drop of either essential oil with 1 teaspoon of honey and
place in a glass. Fill glass with warm water, mixing contents well.
Sip slowly.

Nervous Tension

ESSENTIAL OILS
Chamomile, marjoram, lavender
TREATMENT
Bath. Massage. Air spray. Oil burner.

Nipples, Sore

ESSENTIAL OILS

Chamomile

TREATMENT

Massage the following cream into the nipples daily during pregnancy and after your baby is born. Wash the nipples thoroughly before breast-feeding to remove any surplus cream.

Nipple Cream

30ml (1fl oz) olive or canola oil
1 teaspoon wheat germ oil
½ teaspoon carrot oil
120g (approx. 4oz) Copha (hydrogenated coconut oil cooking fat)
40 drops chamomile oil

Melt the olive or canola, wheat germ and carrot oils and Copha together over a gentle heat. Remove from heat and allow to cool slightly. Add the essential oil and beat well, continuing to beat until mixture is cold. Pot up in a dark-coloured glass jar.

Premenstrual Syndrome (PMS), Nerves and Mood Swings

ESSENTIAL OILS

Chamomile, geranium, marjoram

TREATMENT

Bath. Massage. Air spray. Oil burner.

Premenstrual Syndrome, Water Retention

ESSENTIAL OILS

Fennel, juniper, rosemary

TREATMENT

Massage. Bath.

Psoriasis

ESSENTIAL OILS

Bergamot, lavender

TREATMENT

Facial steam (if problem is on face). Bath. Add 6 drops of mixed oils to 1 tablespoon of sweet almond oil. Use to massage on troubled spots.

Rashes

ESSENTIAL OILS

Chamomile, lavender, tea tree

TREATMENT

Ointment. Baths. Compresses.

Rheumatism

ESSENTIAL OILS

Juniper, pine, rosemary

TREATMENT

Baths. Massage with Massage Cream or Oil.

Ringworm and Scabies

ESSENTIAL OILS

Tea tree, myrrh, lavender

TREATMENT

Ointment. Tea tree oil, applied neat.

Scalds, Minor

ESSENTIAL OILS

Lavender

TREATMENT

Hold scalded area under cold water for up to 10 minutes. Smooth neat lavender oil directly onto scald.

Scar Tissue

ESSENTIAL OILS

Lavender, myrrh

TREATMENT

1 drop of each essential oil in 2 teaspoons of wheat germ oil;
massage daily for as long as necessary.

Shock

ESSENTIAL OILS

Chamomile, peppermint, lavender

TREATMENT

Inhalation. Bath. Massage

Snake Bites

ESSENTIAL OILS

Lavender

TREATMENT

Try to identify the snake. Flood puncture wound with lavender oil.
Bind limb firmly but not tightly with anything available. Keep
patient calm and still. Seek medical help immediately.

Spider Bites

ESSENTIAL OILS

Lavender

TREATMENT

Add 5 drops of oil to 1 teaspoon of vinegar. Dab on bite every four
hours, or more often if needed. If you suspect that the spider was a
poisonous variety, go straight to hospital, dabbing the wound
constantly with neat lavender oil until hospital treatment begins.

Sprains and Strains

ESSENTIAL OILS

Chamomile, lavender, rosemary

TREATMENT

Cold Compress. Massage Cream or Oil.

Stiffness of Muscles or Joints

ESSENTIAL OILS
Black pepper, lavender, rosemary
TREATMENT
Massage, using Massage Cream or Oil. Bath.

Sunburn

ESSENTIAL OILS
Lavender
TREATMENT
Cool bath. Gently smooth Massage Oil or Cream onto the
affected area.

Throat, Sore

ESSENTIAL OILS
Clary sage, lavender, geranium
TREATMENT
Inhalation. Gargle.

Thrush

ESSENTIAL OILS
Cedarwood, lavender, tea tree
TREATMENT
Add 1 drop of each essential oil to 1 tablespoon of yoghurt and 1
teaspoon of water. Use as a douche.

Tonsillitis

ESSENTIAL OILS
Bergamot, hyssop, thyme
TREATMENT
Inhalation. Gargle.

Travel Sickness

ESSENTIAL OILS

Peppermint

TREATMENT

Mix 1 drop with 1 teaspoon of honey in a glass of warm water
and sip slowly.

Varicose Veins

ESSENTIAL OILS

Bergamot, cypress, lemon

TREATMENT

Cold Compress, using 6 drops of mixed essential oils in
2 teaspoons of witch hazel.

Warts and Verrucae

ESSENTIAL OILS

Tea tree

TREATMENT

Drop neat oil onto wart or verruca.

Wasp Stings

ESSENTIAL OILS

Lavender

TREATMENT

Add 4 drops of oil to 1 teaspoon of vinegar. Dab on wound to
counteract the alkaline poison of the sting and to reduce pain and
swelling. Repeat hourly, or as often as needed.

Wounds

ESSENTIAL OILS

Chamomile, lavender, tea tree

TREATMENT

Wound Wash. Dry dressing with a few drops of lavender or tea
tree oil on the pad. Ointment.

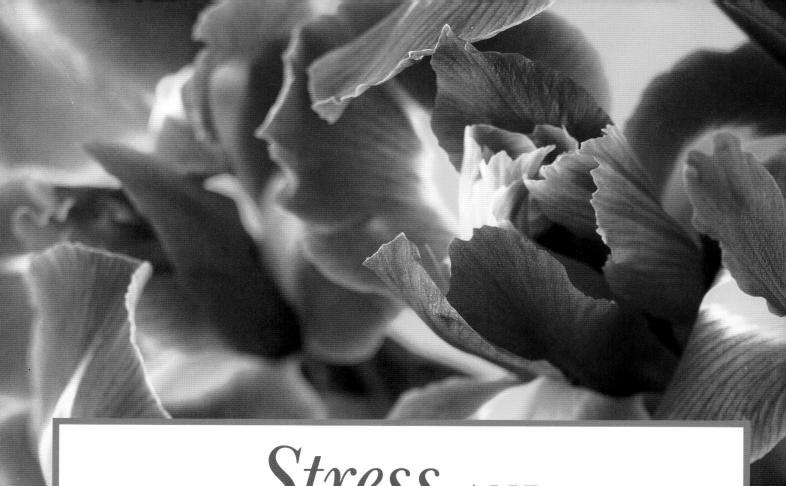

Stress AND Relaxation

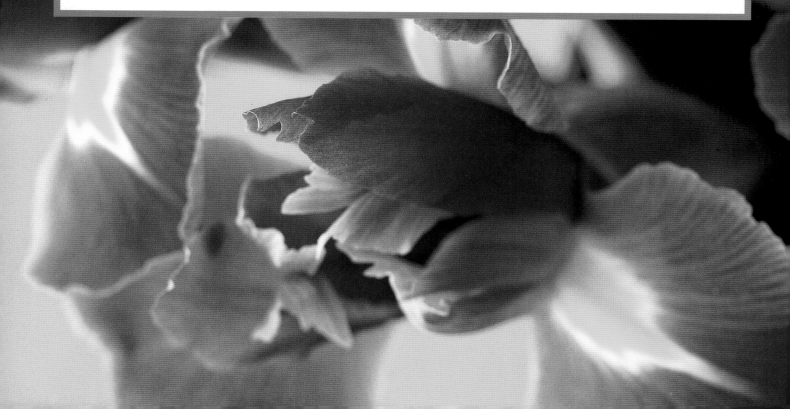

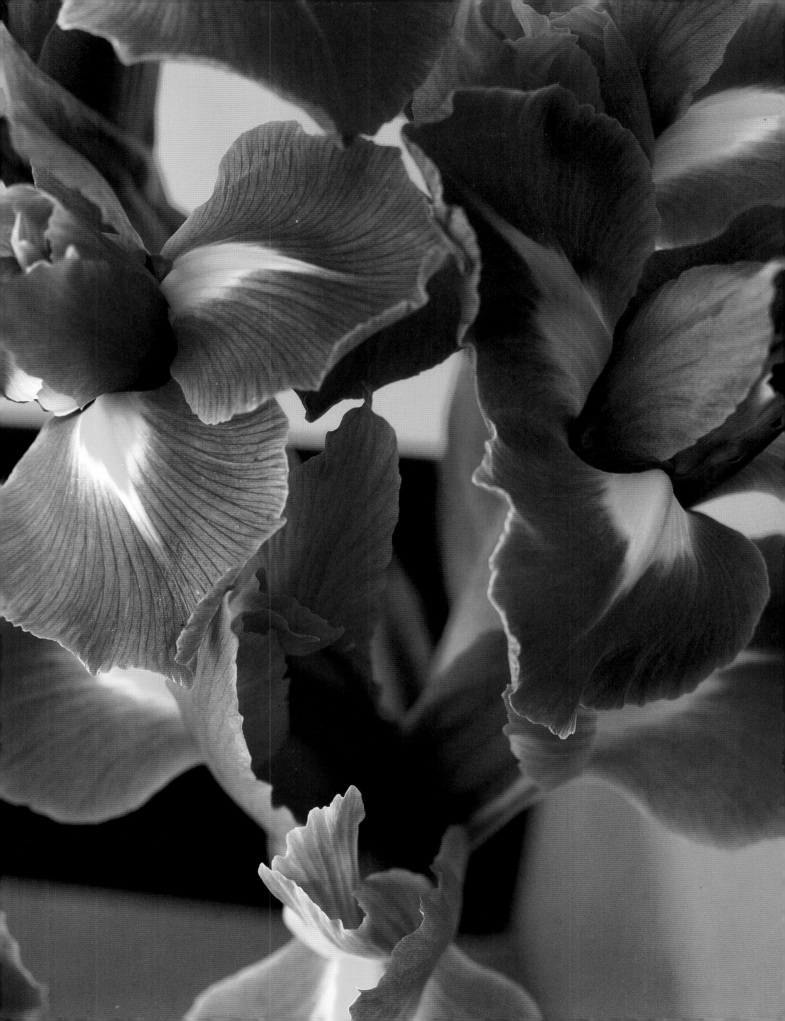

Essential Oils
for Stress Relief

Essential oils are one of the most powerful and precious resources we have on this planet. They are a delightful, sweet-smelling and natural alternative to 'used and abused' drugs, such as Valium. While I would never suggest that a person should discontinue use of prescribed medication, it is often possible to use the essential oils in conjunction with other treatment and eventually, under supervision, to use only essential oils.

This chapter is about stress relief and relaxation, and about some of the ways in which aromatherapy can help to alleviate or prevent stressful situations. For instance, if I am writing to a deadline (which always seems to happen and which I secretly enjoy!), I become aware of my potential physical and mental stress levels. My beautiful and special essential oils are always with me to ensure my welfare. I have an oil burner gently steaming on my desk to look after my mind and emotions, an hourly air spray ensures that positive ions are dispersed, and an after-bath or shower rub with aromatic massage oils counters any muscle stiffness.

It is always better to deal with stressful situations before they become chronic. By allowing essential oils to become part of your life, you will be able to use them as part of a strategy to control any stressful situation in the most relaxed and pleasant way possible. I hope that you will gain some insights from the suggestions in this book, and that it will help you to enjoy life to the full. Rather than letting stress rule and possibly destroy your life, it is my aim to suggest ways in which you can control stress.

What is Stress?

Stress probably began for you today when the alarm clock rang and you opened your eyes. Many people feel that, from this moment on, they are under stress.

The most important step is to identify the type of stress. There are two main types: eustress and dystress.

Sometimes when under stress one can feel like this nut—ready to crack!

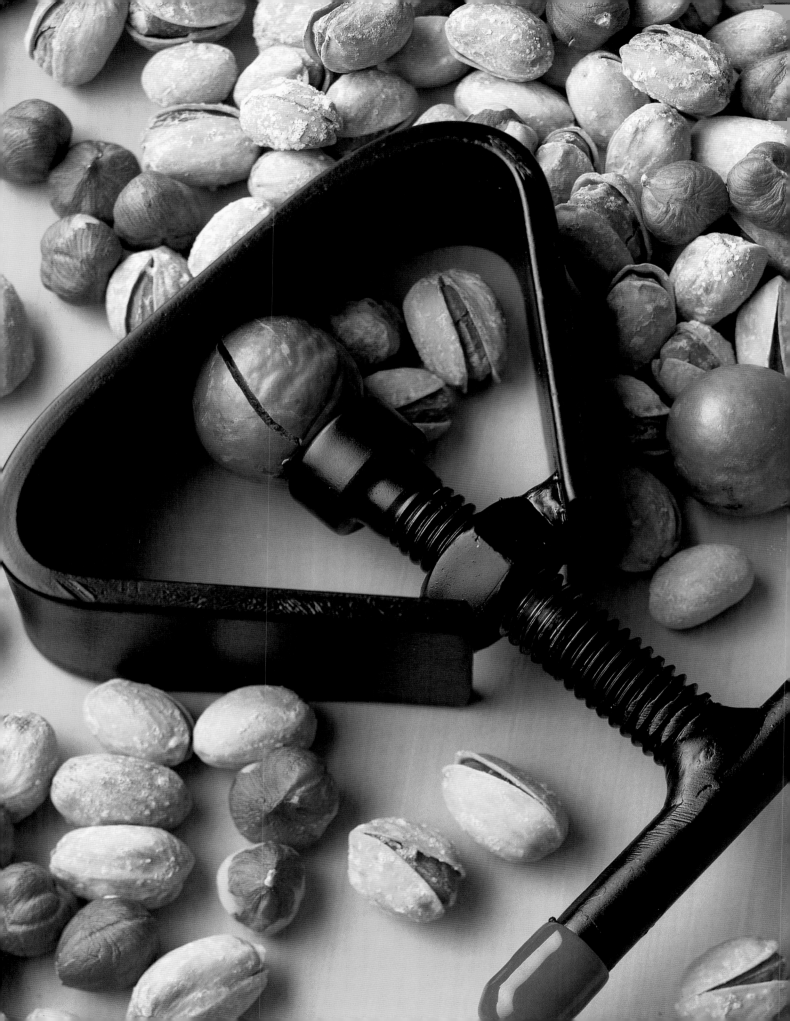

Eustress is the healthy, exhilarating stress which adds sparkle to our lives. We need eustress in order to function and to be alert. It has a beginning, a middle and, most importantly, an end. It is the stress which takes us through a busy and productive day and which, if all our work and play comes to a satisfactory conclusion, is dissipated when we settle down for the evening or go to bed. The chemical changes which take place in our bodies when we are under eustress reverse to a normal, relaxed and healthy state during rest periods.

Dystress (distress) is unhealthy, unresolved stress that is emotionally and physically damaging. The stress chemicals which our bodies produce in stressful situations, such as adrenalin, are not dispersed and can cause high blood pressure, angina, excess cholesterol, stomach ulcers, colitis, cancer, migraine, back problems, depression and nervous breakdowns.

Dystress may be caused by several things: loss or possible loss of a job; loss of a loved one; relationship problems; problems with your children; a too-heavy workload with no end in sight; friction with neighbours or workmates; over-achieving; chronic shortage of money; loneliness; illness; and chemical stress from synthetic materials, pesticides, traffic fumes, television and food additives, to name just a few.

Symptoms of Stress

If you have some or all of the following symptoms, your stress and tension levels are possibly quite severe and need to be addressed before a 'burn out' stage is reached:

- No enthusiasm for work, play, family or friends.
- Finding it difficult to laugh, and getting upset very easily.
- A feeling of impending doom hanging over you.
- Backaches, headaches or stomach aches.
- An inability to sleep, or waking up in the morning feeling just as anxious and as tired as when you went to bed.

It is vital for the sake of your health to resolve these symptoms. There are many methods to relieve stress, depending on the type of problem being experienced. For instance: meditation, the use of essential oils, conflict resolution therapy, counselling, exercise, nutrition, and adequate good quality sleep.

Essential Oils for Stress Relief and Relaxation

Bergamot
(Citrus bergamia)

Lightens depression, anxiety and nervousness by calming, refreshing and lifting the spirit. Allays anger and frustration.
CAUTION: Not to be used on the skin before exposure to sunlight as it may cause pigmentation.

Cedarwood
(Juniperus virginiana; Cedrus atlantica)

Soothes the nervous and over-excitable person. Softens and 'mellows' those with selfish, unyielding, stiff-necked attitudes. Allows the release of mental strain and stress. Gently soothes and helps those with depression and insomnia. A valuable oil for use during meditation.
CAUTION: Not to be used during pregnancy. An irritant to some types of sensitive skin.

Chamomile
(Anthemis nobilis; Matricaria chamomilla)

Soothes the nervously over-excitable person. Relieves mental strain and stress. Relieves depression, anxiety and insomnia. Calms anger and allows us to see problems in perspective.

Clary Sage
(Salvia sclarea)

Allays stress, anxiety and depression. Gives clarity and calmness in situations where there is panic, and allows us the opportunity to deal with the cause. In small doses, clary sage can alleviate hysteria and paranoia.
CAUTION: Large doses can cause headaches and poisoning. Not to be used during pregnancy.

Cypress
(Cupressus sempervirens)

Eases the pain of loss or separation from loved ones, and allows us to 'let go with love'. Lightens the burden of gloominess and introspection. Calms irritability and anger.

Frankincense
(Boswellia thurifera; B. carterii)

Calms and quietens those who nervously 'gush and babble'. Allows anxious and obsessive personalities to drop past hurts (either real or imagined) and to get things in perspective. A spiritual type of oil which enables us to live in the present. A valuable oil to use during meditation.

CAUTION: Can be very irritating if used directly on the skin.

Geranium
(Pelargonium graveolens)

A very feminine oil, particularly suitable for menopausal depression. Promotes harmony and grace. Quells depression, anxiety and stress. May be useful for treating manic depression.

Grapefruit
(Citrus paradisi)

Lifts and revives the spirits and, by so doing, eases depression, nervous headaches, nervous exhaustion and performance-related stress. May help to relieve migraine. May also be useful for manic depressive states.

Jasmine
(Jasminum officinale; J. grandiflorum)

Uplifts and transforms; jasmine will counter listlessness, indifference and apathy, and give confidence. An important oil to arouse those who are suffering from deep depression. Very useful for those in the caring professions, such as nursing, who are suffering from 'burn out'. A useful and deeply relaxing oil for men who are insecure about their sexuality.

CAUTION: Not to be used during pregnancy until labour has begun.

Toilet water is a lovely way to apply essential oils

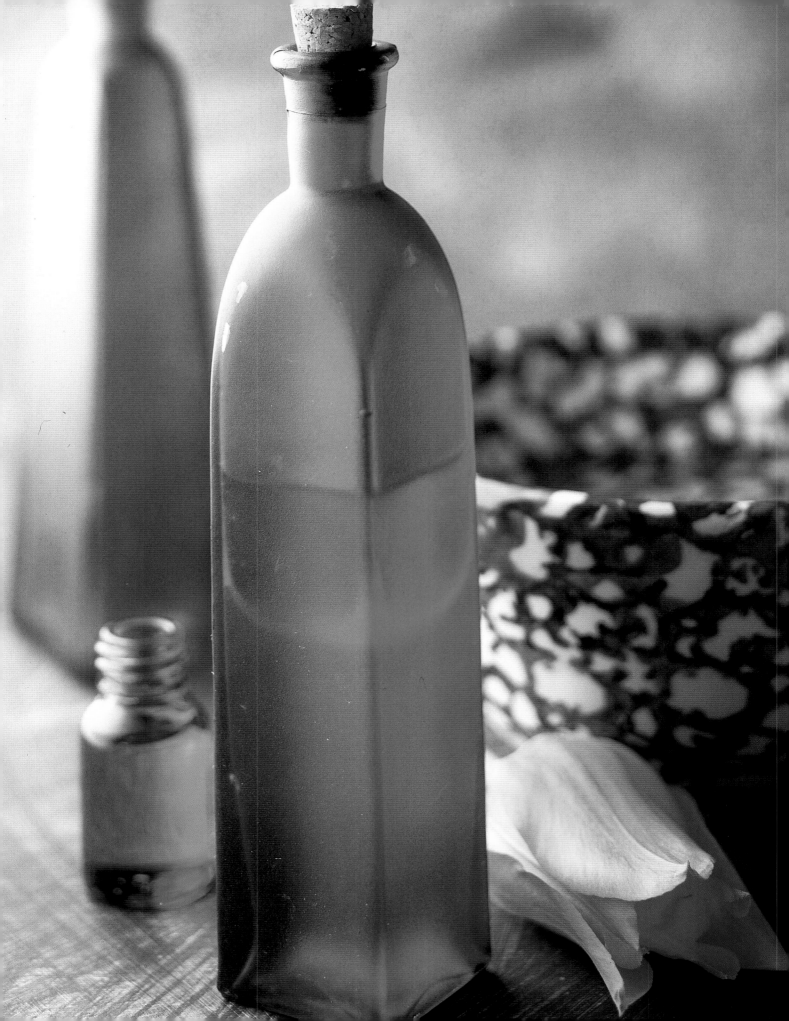

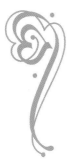

Lavender
(Lavandula angustifolia; L. officinalis)

Possibly the most important essential oil. Lavender balances the emotions on every level, and can create calm from chaos. May be helpful for those who suffer from depression, headaches, insomnia, manic depression, nervous tension, premenstrual syndrome (PMS), shock or vertigo.

CAUTION: May be contra-indicated for those who have low blood pressure.

Lemon
(Citrus limonum)

A must for the student, office worker or computer operator. It clears the mind of sluggishness and apathy, leaving you feeling alert, bright and clear-headed.

Mandarin
(Citrus reticulata)

This oil is included because its non-toxic, non-irritant properties make it very suitable for pregnant women, the elderly and children. It is gentle, refreshing and calming, and is particularly useful for treating insomnia, restlessness and tension.

Marjoram
(Origanum majorana)

Consoles, heals and strengthens a grief-stricken or lonely heart and brings peace. Calms those who are over-excitable, and relieves anxiety and trauma. Helpful for easing nervous headaches, migraine, fainting attacks and insomnia.

CAUTION: Not to be used during pregnancy.

Peppermint
(Mentha piperita)

Promotes mental clarity and positive vibrations. Relieves the symptoms of shock and hysteria, such as fainting, vertigo and palpitations. Helps to disperse anger and depression.

CAUTION: Not to be used during pregnancy. No more than 1% dilution to be used.

Rosemary
(Rosmarinus officinalis)

Lifts the spirits and mind from apathy. Clears that 'woolly' feeling from the brain and gives strength and power to thought processes. Relieves depression and mental and nervous exhaustion and other stress-related disorders.

CAUTION: Not to be used during pregnancy or by people with epilepsy.

Sandalwood
(Santalum album)

Traditionally known as 'the meditator's oil', as it is uplifting and spiritual. Relieves tension, anxiety, insomnia and obsessive behaviour. A beautiful oil to comfort the dying.

Ylang-ylang
(Cananga odorata)

Creates a feeling of tranquillity and calm, making for an environment in which frustrating or unpleasant jobs or unwelcome encounters can be tackled. Counters depression. Eases anger, fear, panic, nervousness and tension related to sexual matters.

Anti-stress Treatments

Flowers from Lisa Milasas

Air Sprays

Air sprays are useful for creating a light aura of perfume in a room. Avoid spraying directly onto polished furniture or near fish tanks. The sprays may be made in a variety of sizes, ranging from little pocket-sized spray flasks up to 300ml (10fl oz) spray bottles, depending on the use you are going to make of them. The basic recipe below may be adapted to different sized containers.

Basic Airspray

40–80 drops essential oil
50ml ($1^2/3$fl oz) vodka or apple cider vinegar
250ml (8fl oz) water

Dissolve the essential oil in the vodka or vinegar. Add the water and shake well to mix. Shake the bottle before each use.

Aromatic Bath

Quiet, warm and peaceful…baths are an ideal way of using essential oils to alleviate stress, insomnia, depression and other stress-related problems. In fact, it is very difficult to lie in warm, beautifully scented water and remain tense or miserable!

Make sure that you have plenty of time and that you are not going to be disturbed. The room should be warm and not too brightly lit (candles are ideal) and you should have something comfortable to rest your head on. When dealing with stress-related problems, remember that the bath water should never be too hot —'comfort' is the key word for this experience!

Mix the selected essential oils with a tablespoon or so of full cream milk. This ensures that the oils disperse completely in the water. Add and 'swoosh' the water thoroughly, climb in and relax.

Breathe slowly and gently. As you breathe in, feel the aromatic vapours entering every cell of your body and mind, collecting all negative, tense, tired feelings into a grey mist. As you breathe out, imagine the grey mist being breathed out, too. You could also use the 'One' meditation (at the end of this chapter) at this time.

Remain in the bath for at least 20 minutes; top up with more warm water if necessary. After the bath, imagine all the tension and negative feelings running down the drain with the bath water.

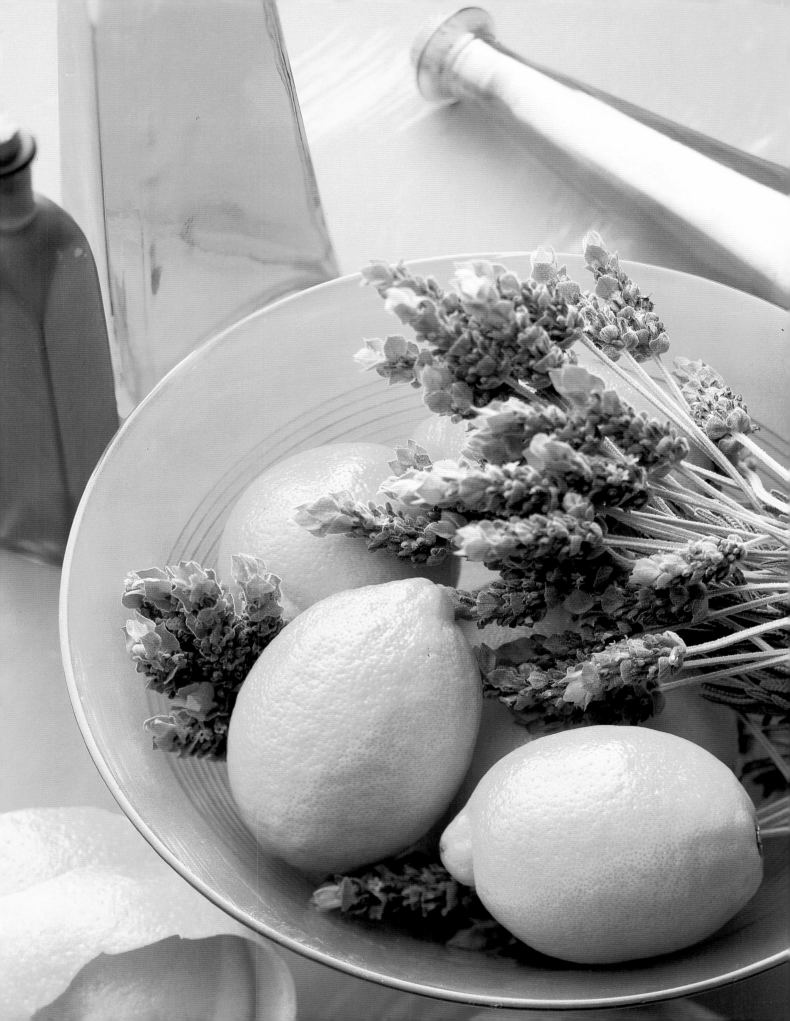

Toilet Water

Toilet water may be used as an after-bath or shower splash, or as a refreshing skin treat during the day. The essential oils can be chosen from any relevant recipes throughout the book.

Basic Toilet Water

1 tablespoon vodka (less 1 teaspoon)
2 tablespoons witch hazel
2 tablespoons purified water
$^1/_2$ teaspoon glycerine
15 drops essential oil

Mix all ingredients in a 100ml ($3^1/_3$fl oz) bottle. Shake well. Leave for 4 days to blend thoroughly.

Massage

Massage is a powerful way to dispel stress and tension. The essential oils are absorbed through the skin and into the blood stream, and from there they influence all the body systems. The aromas enter the olfactory system to reach the innermost parts of the brain, where they influence thinking and feeling processes. The other benefit to be obtained from a massage is that of touch —we feel cherished when someone lays their hands on us in a caring and therapeutic way.

Essential Oil Blends

If you do not have one of the oils specified in a recipe, you may substitute another from the following list.

Sometimes, a particular blend may not seem to exactly 'fit' the way you are feeling. Make up your own blend, using the emotions and conditions detailed below as a guide.

Also, it is not always very satisfactory to use all the oils suggested for one condition. Instead, try to choose just one or two for the main problem, along with another one or two which balance the blend.

ANGER
ESSENTIAL OILS Bergamot, chamomile, cypress, peppermint, ylang-ylang

ANXIETY
ESSENTIAL OILS Bergamot, chamomile, clary sage, frankincense, geranium, lavender, mandarin, marjoram, sandalwood

APATHY
ESSENTIAL OILS Grapefruit, jasmine, lavender, lemon, rosemary

BALANCER (MOODS)
ESSENTIAL OILS Lavender, geranium, jasmine

'BURN OUT'
ESSSENTIAL OILS Jasmine, lavender

CALMING
ESSENTIAL OILS Bergamot, cedarwood, clary sage, frankincense, jasmine, lavender, mandarin, marjoram, sandalwood, ylang-ylang

CHILDREN (GENERAL)
ESSENTIAL OILS 1 wk–2 mths: Lavender, chamomile; 2 mths–2 yrs: Chamomile, geranium, lavender, mandarin, spearmint

DEPRESSION
ESSENTIAL OILS Bergamot, cedarwood, clary sage, chamomile, frankincense, geranium, grapefruit, jasmine, lavender, mandarin, peppermint, rosemary

EMOTIONAL STRESS
ESSENTIAL OILS Ylang-ylang

EXCITABILITY
ESSENTIAL OILS Cedarwood, chamomile, lavender, mandarin, marjoram, ylang-ylang

FAINTING
ESSENTIAL OILS Lavender, marjoram, peppermint

FRIGIDITY
ESSENTIAL OILS Clary sage, ylang-ylang

FRUSTRATION
ESSENTAIL OILS Bergamot, lavender

GRIEF
ESSENTIAL OILS Cypress, marjoram, sandalwood

GUILT
ESSENTIAL OILS Chamomile, clary sage, sandalwood

HYSTERIA
ESSENTIAL OILS Clary sage, peppermint

INSOMNIA
ESSENTIAL OILS Cedarwood, chamomile, lavender, mandarin, marjoram, sandalwood

IRRITABILITY
ESSENTIAL OIL Cypress

LISTLESSNESS
ESSENTIAL OILS Geranium, jasmine, lavender

MANIC DEPRESSION
ESSENTIAL OILS Geranium, grapefruit, lavender

MEDITATION
ESSENTIAL OILS Cedarwood, frankincense, sandalwood

MENOPAUSE
ESSENTIAL OILS Bergamot, clary sage, geranium, jasmine, rose

MENTAL DULLNESS
ESSENTIAL OILS Lemon, peppermint, rosemary

MENTAL STRESS
ESSENTIAL OILS Cedarwood, chamomile, rosemary

MIGRAINE
ESSENTIAL OILS Grapefruit, marjoram

NEGATIVE THOUGHTS
ESSENTIAL OILS Orange, peppermint

NERVOUS EXHAUSTION
ESSENTIAL OILS Grapefruit, lavender, rosemary, ylang-ylang

NERVOUS HEADACHE
ESSENTIAL OILS Grapefruit, lavender, marjoram

NERVOUSNESS (JITTERS)
ESSENTIAL OILS Bergamot, frankincense, geranium, lavender

OBSESSIVENESS
ESSENTIAL OILS Frankincense, sandalwood

PANIC
ESSENTIAL OILS Clary sage, ylang-ylang

PARANOIA
ESSENTAIL OIL Clary sage

PRE-MENSTRUAL SYNDROME (PMS)
ESSENTIAL OILS Bergamot, chamomile, clary sage, geranium, grapefruit, jasmine, lavender

RESTLESSNESS
ESSENTIAL OILS Marjoram, ylang-ylang

SEXUALITY (INSECURITY)
ESSENTIAL OILS Clary sage, jasmine, sandalwood, ylang-ylang

SHOCK
ESSENTIAL OILS Lavender, peppermint

SLUGGISHNESS (MENTAL)
ESSENTIAL OILS Lemon, grapefruit

TRAUMA
ESSENTIAL OILS Lavender, marjoram

VERTIGO
ESSENTIAL OILS Lavender, peppermint

NOTE: Consult the 'Blending Guide' (in Chapter 1) and 'Anti-stress Treatments' (this chapter) for methods and quantities to use in the recipes which follow.

Cushion from Art Park, jug from Dinosaur Designs, flowers from Lisa Milasas

Keep the Calming Blend air spray on hand

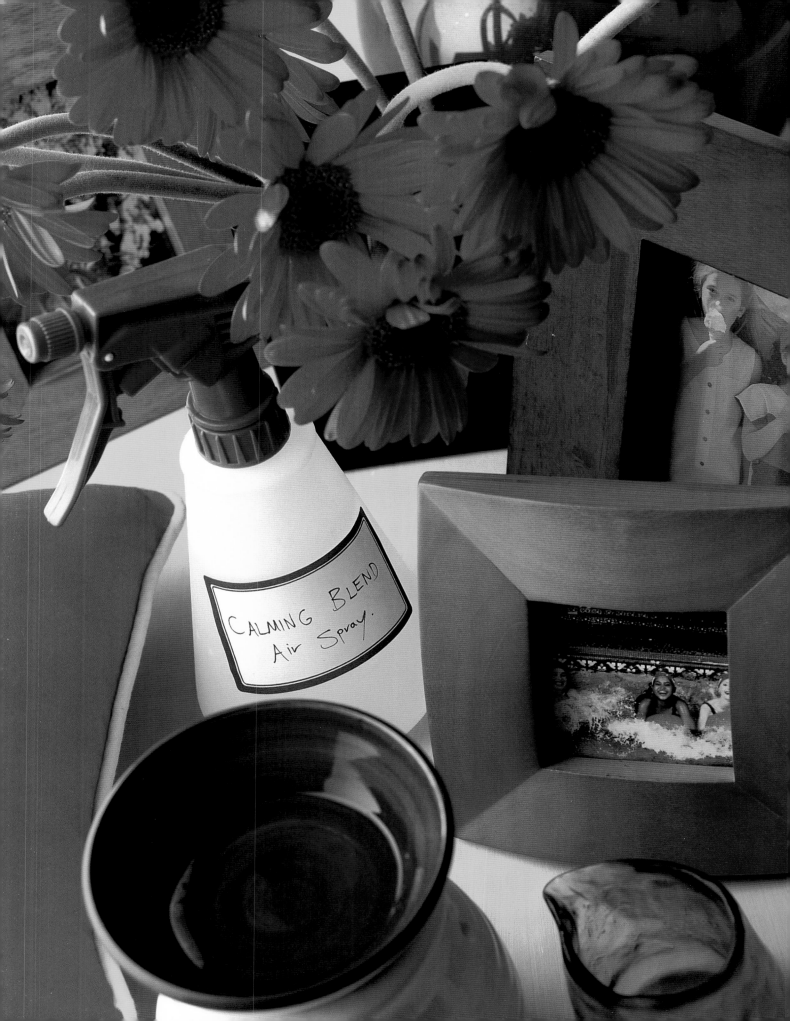

Stress in the Home

Your home should be your haven. However it is often, through a variety of circumstances, a most stressful arena; instead of welcoming you home, it can be like stepping onto a battlefield!

Try to come to this arrangement with your family: that no one complains about their day until half an hour after the last person has arrived home. During this half hour, slip your shoes off, have a cup of tea or a glass of wine or whatever relaxes you, and put your feet up in your bedroom or in the garden. If everyone does this, they may well forget what they were going to grizzle about!

These days an increasing number of people work both in and out of the home. Even if it is from choice, this can become excessively stressful, particularly if the extra work is taken on from economic necessity. It is important in such circumstances to have regular (maybe weekly) family meetings to sort out areas of dissatisfaction, and also to praise each other for kindnesses or triumphs which may have transpired since the previous week. It is sad but true that it is easier to be nice to strangers than to members of our own family!

Each member of the family needs to share part of the work load. Even little children can do simple jobs, and even the smallest job done well and regularly helps to ease the strain. Swap the jobs around every few weeks to prevent boredom or a feeling of being 'put upon'.

Use essential oils as part of your strategy to restore or maintain your home as a safe, calm and loving place, where you can release anxieties, regain strength of purpose and allow the hectic world to recede until you are ready to 'face the pace' once more. The whole family will benefit from the use of essential oils in the home and also from the feeling that something positive and happy is being created for all, from the tiny newborn baby to great-grandparent. It is astonishing how your spirits can lift when some forward movement is made and the members of a household realise that they love each other and want to look after each other.

Every part of your home can receive the benefits of essential oils. There are several different ways of diffusing the oils into the air. The three most important are:

- Air sprays and oil burners that can be used to create a general calming influence on family members in the living rooms and bedrooms. These sprays and burners can also contain oils to soothe and safeguard during times when illness threatens or is present.

- Baths that are deeply therapeutic and stress-reducing—even the most frantic baby is often soothed and calmed by being placed in warm, scented water.

- Massage. This can be a loving, tender and non-threatening way for family members to draw close to each other. Older people may feel timid about a body massage, but will gain immense pleasure and benefit from a foot or shoulder massage.

The following recipes will be a guide to some ways in which you can employ the oils in your home. Oils may be substituted by looking at the 'Essential Oil Blends' list previously this chapter.

Living Room

Happy Families

This blend counters depression, and is joyful and uplifting.

2 teaspoons lavender oil
2 teaspoons grapefruit oil
$^1/_2$ teaspoon bergamot oil
$^1/_2$ teaspoon sandalwood oil

Mix all the oils in a 25ml (approx. 1fl oz) bottle. Shake well. Leave for 4 days to blend thoroughly.

Suggested uses:
- Air spray or oil burner, on radiators, on wood for the fire.
- A few drops on a light bulb before switching the light on.
- This blend is also good in the bath, for after shower use, and in massage oils.

Pillow slip covers from Art Park, cup from Dinosaur Designs, flowers from Lisa Milasas

TIP

Cooking a meal at the end of a long hard day can either contribute to your stress levels, or it can be a time for gradually unwinding, laughing and talking about the experiences of the day. Encourage the whole family to participate in food preparation—not as a chore but as a learning and sharing experience.

Kitchens

Citrus Fresh

Use this blend for a calm, cheerful atmosphere during the preparation of food.

> *2 teaspoons lemon oil*
> *1 teaspoon bergamot oil*
> *1 teaspoon grapefruit oil*
> *½ teaspoon sandalwood oil*
> *½ teaspoon lavender oil*

Mix all the oils in a 25ml (approx. 1fl oz) bottle. Shake well. Leave for 4 days to blend thoroughly.

Suggested uses:
- In an air spray or an oil burner before cooking begins.
- Sprinkle on a damp cloth and use to wipe work surfaces.

Bedrooms

More than all the other rooms in the house, the bedrooms should be restful. Lighting and colours need to be low-key and perfumes soft, conducive to companionable talk, love-making and sleep. Children need a feeling of security and privacy in their bedrooms.

All too often the bedroom can become a battleground, as parents often wait until they are alone in the bedroom to air their grievances. Have disagreements in the car (in the garage!) or down the bottom of the garden, but not in the bedroom.

Sometimes a partner has a feeling of sexual inadequacy or timidity which can lead to bitterness and guilt or blame. If the problem is a too-demanding partner, a spray containing marjoram oil might help to quell the excessive ardour!

Adults often imagine that they have a monopoly on worry and that children are (or should be) completely carefree. I remember that when I was a little girl, a rolled-up carpet in the corner of my bedroom became a stalking monster as soon as the light went out . Fortunately, my mother believed me (or said that she did) and found somewhere else to store the carpet. Examination nerves, performance-related stress in sport, peer group pressure, acne and puppy fat, along with many more real or imagined fears can make life very difficult for young people.

Bedrooms are the ideal place to use essential oils

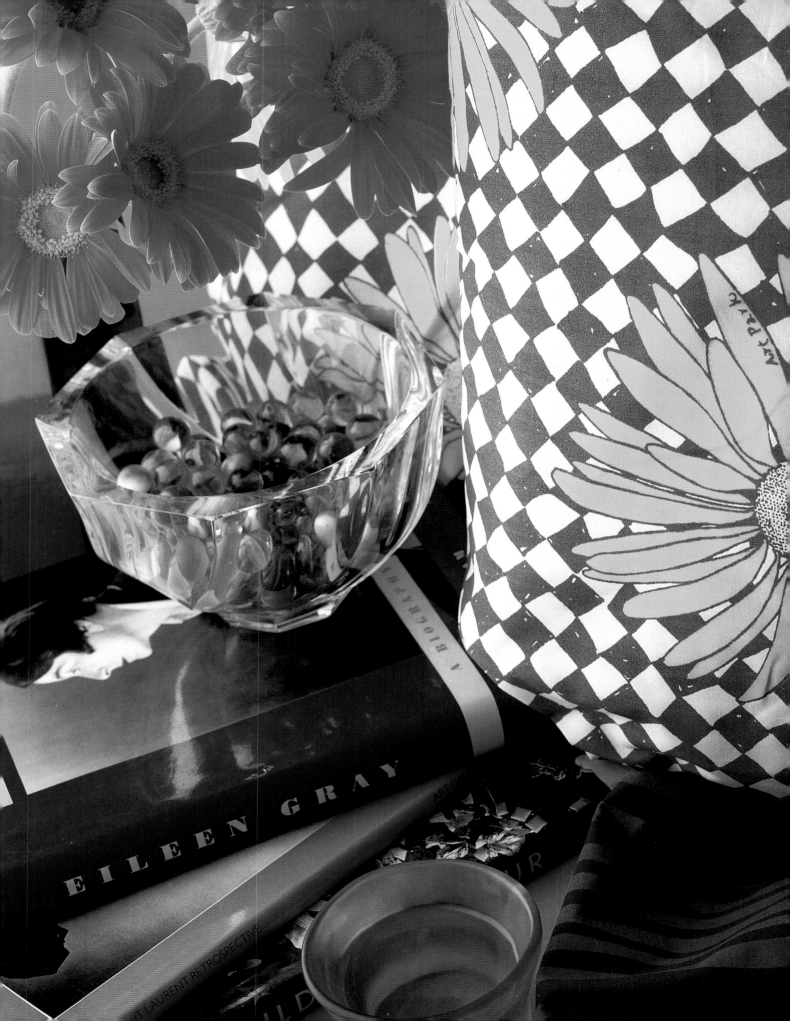

EILEEN GRAY

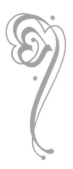

The following oil blends will help to create a bedroom oasis.

The Restful Bedroom for Adults

2 teaspoons bergamot oil
1 teaspoon lavender oil
1 teaspoon mandarin oil
1 teaspoon ylang-ylang oil

Mix all the oils in a 25ml (approx. 1fl oz) bottle. Shake well. Leave for 4 days to blend thoroughly.

Suggested uses:
- Use in an air spray a few minutes before retiring, or in an oil burner (not near curtains, bedclothes or inflammable materials).
- Sprinkle a few drops on cottonwool balls and tuck under pillows or under the bed.
- Make a flat sachet out of 2 handkerchiefs sewn together, sprinkle with 1–3 drops of the blend, slip inside the pillowcase.

The Romantic Bedroom

2 teaspoons sandalwood oil
1½ teaspoons clary sage oil
1 teaspoon ylang-ylang oil
40 drops jasmine or neroli oil

Mix all the oils in a 25ml (approx. 1fl oz) bottle. Shake well. Leave for 4 days to blend thoroughly.

Suggested uses:
- See The Restful Bedroom for Adults.

Sleeping Easy

1 teaspoon chamomile oil
2 teaspoons lavender oil
1 teaspoon marjoram oil
1 teaspoon clary sage oil

Mix all the oils in a 25ml (approx. 1fl oz) bottle. Shake well. Leave for 4 days to blend thoroughly.

Suggested uses:
- See The Restful Bedroom for Adults.

For Tired Minds

2 teaspoons geranium oil
1 teaspoon lavender oil
1 teaspoon ylang-ylang oil
½ teaspoon cedarwood oil
½ teaspoon sandalwood oil

Mix all the oils in a 25ml (approx. 1fl oz) bottle. Shake well. Leave for 4 days to blend thoroughly.

Suggested uses:
• See The Restful Bedroom for Adults.

For Tired Nerves

2 teaspoons sandalwood or frankincense oil
1 teaspoon lavender oil
1 teaspoon ylang-ylang oil
½ teaspoon bergamot oil
½ teaspoon cedarwood oil

Mix all the oils in a 25ml (approx. 1fl oz) bottle. Shake well. Leave for 4 days to blend thoroughly.

Suggested uses:
• See The Restful Bedroom for Adults.

Babies (2 days–2 years)

80ml (2⅔fl oz) sweet almond oil
1 tablespoon olive oil
5 drops chamomile oil
8 drops lavender oil

Mix the oils in a 100ml (3⅓fl oz) bottle. Shake well. Leave 4 days.

Suggested uses:
• Float a drop of this oil blend in a bowl of warm water under the cot, or use it in an air spray just before bedtime.
• Babies love to be massaged. Massaging creates strong bonding and also has a calming effect on a baby who is fretful or suffering from colic. The combination of these oils and a gentle massage can often ensure a good night's sleep for baby.

Children (2 years–teens)

This oil blend will help to disperse the worries of the day and create a serene and peaceful atmosphere for sound sleep.

2 teaspoons geranium oil
2 teaspoons lavender oil
1 teaspoon chamomile oil

Mix all the oils in a 25ml (approx. 1fl oz) bottle. Shake well. Leave for 4 days to blend thoroughly.

Suggested uses:
- 4 to 8 drops (depending on the age) can be mixed with 1 tablespoon of vegetable oil and sprinkled on the surface of the bathwater after the bath has been run. 'Swoosh' the water well.
- Mix up to 20 drops (depending on age) with 100ml ($3\frac{1}{3}$fl oz) of sweet almond oil and use as a massage oil.
- Float a few drops of the blend in a bowl of hot water and place under or near the bed.
- Put 2 to 3 drops on cottonwool balls; tuck one under the pillow and place 2 or 3 around the room.

The Restful Bedroom for Children

Children love the warm and friendly smell of mandarin. This is an excellent blend to help students to feel positive and happy.

2 teaspoons lavender oil
2 teaspoons geranium oil
1 teaspoon mandarin oil

Mix all the oils in a 25ml (approx. 1fl oz) bottle. Shake well. Leave for 4 days to blend thoroughly.

Suggested uses:
- Put a few drops of the blend on cottonwool balls and place them in pockets, satchels and desks.
- A drop or two can be put on a tissue or handkerchief and sniffed when needed.
- Include the blend in a little bottle of massage oil, which can be carried and used to rub on pulse points.
- Mix the blend up as a toilet water for spraying on neck, arms and legs; it can be carried to school in a spray bottle or atomiser.

Children also need the benefits of aromatherapy

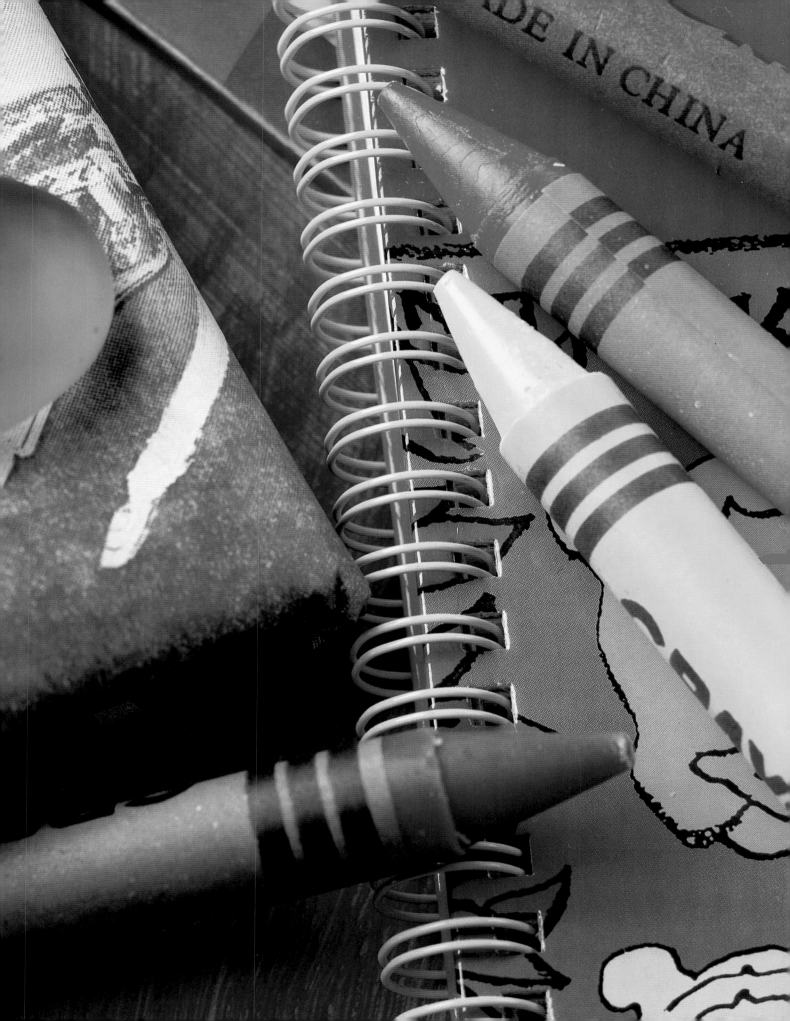

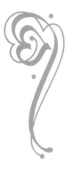

On the Way to Work and School

Well! We all know what a drama this can be, so I will not dwell on the traumas which can erupt as soon as you all leave the house. You can help to avoid this sort of stress and create a happy, positive and calm atmosphere with the following suggestions:

- Mix equal amounts of peppermint and lavender oil in a small dropper bottle and store in a little box or bag with some cottonwool balls. Use a drop or two of this oil blend on a few of the balls and tuck them around the car — the dashboard, the rear window ledge, on top of the sun visors and under or down the sides of seats are all good spots.
- Put a drop or two on a handkerchief or tissue for each person, for them to sniff as needed.
- When you are waiting at traffic lights or in traffic jams, encourage everyone in the car (including you) to slowly lift their shoulders up to try to touch their ears while breathing in. Let the shoulders flop down and relax as the breath comes out in a long sigh. This is very relaxing, as we hold a great deal of tension in our shoulders and necks.
- Gritting the teeth and jaw on the in-breath and relaxing on the out-breath is another good method of releasing tension.

Getting Ready

Whether you work alone, as I do, or in a busy, noisy office or factory, there are stresses with which one has to contend.

It is important to first sit down and itemise which parts of your day are the most stressful. For instance, do demands from other people interfere with your own work? Do you have too-high expectations of yourself or others? Are you subject to high noise levels, isolation, or being on your feet or on your bottom for excessive lengths of time, and are you in an unhealthily synthetic environment? You will probably be able to add many more stress factors to this list.

I have found that, with a little forethought, many of these stressors can be either reduced or got rid of altogether. We put up with things because that is how they have always been (and, if we are honest, because it is easy to be a martyr).

In conjunction with this reorganisation, make sure that you are using essential oils, eating well, sleeping well, having fun leisure time, and communicating with your family and friends.

The following recipes will help to ensure that your working life becomes easier and more joyful.

Day Break for Girls

The 'smooth you out and perk you up' blend to begin your day.

1 teaspoon bergamot oil
1 teaspoon geranium oil
2 teaspoons lavender oil
40 drops peppermint oil
40 drops clary sage oil

Mix all the oils in a 25ml (approx. 1fl oz) bottle. Shake well. Leave for 4 days to blend thoroughly.

Suggested uses:
- In an after-shower oil rub or in a toilet water splash.
- As a bath oil
- Put 2 drops on a cottonwool ball and tuck it in the front of your bra where the heat of your body will evaporate the oil.
- Put 2 to 3 drops on a cottonwool ball or tissue and tuck it in your handbag or purse to enliven you each time you open it.

Day Break for Guys

Same effects as the one for girls, but a special blend for men.

2 teaspoons bergamot oil
1 teaspoon lemon oil
1 teaspoon rosemary oil
1 teaspoon cedarwood oil

Mix all the oils in a 25ml (approx. 1fl oz) bottle. Shake well. Leave for 4 days to blend thoroughly.

Suggested uses:
- Same as for the girls' blend, except for the bra bit!
- Use in an aftershave toilet water splash.

TIP

Emotional stresses often
require professional help in
order to learn conflict
resolution methods or
assertiveness, but the
essential oils are also an
invaluable aid while you are
coming to grips with such
problems—they really do
smooth the path. Even if
you do not experience
conflict in your day, the oils
will help you to sail
tranquilly through a
power-packed, busy and
demanding schedule.

At the Workplace

It is quite likely that your workplace has airconditioning, computers, synthetic carpets, synthetic furnishings and veneered furniture. These are just a few of the chemical stresses with which we are confronted each day. They are potentially very hazardous to our health but, fortunately, there is quite a lot we can do to counteract them.

Physical stresses involve sitting or standing for long periods of time, using machines or computers and being exposed to other peoples' airborne germs. Take a minute or two to stretch your muscles at least every fifteen to twenty minutes, and make sure that you are adequately protected with a 'bug-buster' essential oil blend if sick people are thoughtless enough to come to work and breathe all over their workmates.

Antibacterial Blend

2 teaspoons lavender oil
1 teaspoon cypress oil
1 teaspoon rosemary oil
1 teaspoon eucalyptus oil

Mix all the oils in a 25ml (approx. 1fl oz) bottle. Shake well. Leave for 4 days to blend thoroughly.

Suggested uses:
• Use in air sprays or in an oil burner on your desk or near your work area.
• Put 2 drops of this oil blend on a handkerchief or tissue and inhale the scent as needed.
• Have a shower or at least a wash midway through your day, followed by a toilet water splash containing this blend to help to disperse the positive ions and increase the negative ion effect.
• Wear clothing made from natural materials.
• Keep a piece of pure wool carpet under your feet, which has been sprayed with a little air spray containing this blend.

Use an air spray or oil burner at the workplace and choose a blend that is pleasant for all those nearby

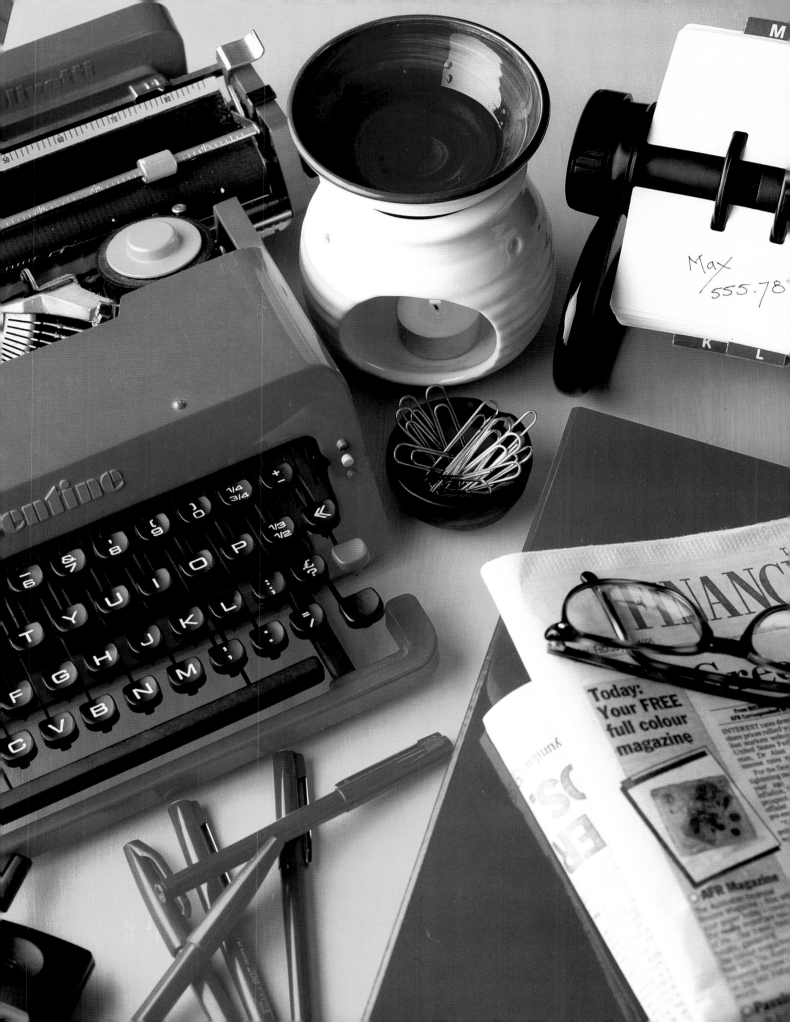

Stale Air Reviver

2 teaspoons lemon oil
1 teaspoon lavender oil
1 teaspoon grapefruit oil
1 teaspoon cypress oil

Mix all the oils in a 25ml (approx. 1fl oz) bottle. Shake well. Leave for 4 days to blend thoroughly.

Suggested uses:
- Adjust the above blend until it suits everyone in your environment, and use in an air spray and oil burner.

Pulse Point Blend for Brain Fatigue

1 tablespoon sweet almond oil
8 drops bergamot oil
8 drops lemon oil
6 drops rosemary oil

Mix all the oils together in a 25ml (approx. 1fl oz) bottle. Shake well before use.

Suggested uses:
- Massage onto temples and forehead, and on pulse points inside wrists and throat. Inhale the perfume.
- Put 2 drops on a tissue or handkerchief and inhale as often as needed.
- This blend can also be made up in a Toilet Water (described previously in this chapter) and used to wipe over the hands, arms and neck to refresh and 'de-stress'.

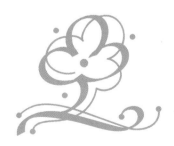

Burn Out

'Burn Out' Blend

Your family and friends have been telling you for weeks, even months, to slow down. However, you felt invincible—or at least you felt that if you did not do all the work yourself the whole universe would grind to a halt! And now? You are so mentally and physically exhausted, you have scarcely enough energy to get up in the morning.

It is not to late to begin to take care of yourself, but quite a lot of lifestyle changes will be needed. Some of these are listed following this recipe.

2 teaspoons lavender oil
1 teaspoon grapefruit oil
1 teaspoon lemon oil
1 teaspoon sandalwood oil

Mix all the oils in a 25ml (approx. 1fl oz) bottle. Shake well. Leave for 4 days to blend thoroughly.

Suggested ways to manage 'burn-out':
- Use the blend in the bath and in massage oils, air sprays, oil burners or in toilet water splashes.
- Lessen your workload.
- Arrange to have a once or twice weekly massage using this 'burn out' blend in the massage oil. If you cannot afford a professional massage, you can 'trade off' with a partner or friend; it is almost as rewarding to give a massage as it is to receive one!
- Eat plenty of fresh, unprocessed food but do not eat if you are upset or over-tired. Wait until you are calmer or your body will not be able to cope with digesting the food.
- Get a minimum of eight hours sleep every night.
- Avoid negative people and situations. Take a rest from reading or watching the news—it will all continue to happen even if you are not monitoring it!
- Allow yourself time to be alone with no demands being made on your time or energy.
- Take some sort of exercise every day, such as walking or swimming, or whatever you enjoy most.
- Do not be embarrassed or afraid to ask for help.
- Learn to meditate.

Sports Stress

Never underestimate the stress created by sport, particularly competitive sport. There is the pre-game stress, with all the worries about being a worthwhile part of the team, and the unresolved stress after the game if you feel that you have failed or could have achieved more.

I must confess to being really perturbed by the stress to which many parents expose their children in this area. I have heard parents offering bribes and even threats in an effort to persuade a child to 'achieve'. Games are supposed to be fun!

Use the following essential oil blends before and after sport and, above all, enjoy the game.

Pre-sport Massage Oil

This massage oil will tone your muscles so that they are ready for the football game, marathon walk, triathlon or whatever. It will also help you to achieve a calm, positive frame of mind.

100ml ($3^{1}/_{3}$fl oz) sweet almond oil, less 1 teaspoon
20 drops rosemary oil
20 drops cypress oil
20 drops lavender oil
10 drops juniper oil

Mix all in a 100ml ($3^{1}/_{3}$fl oz) bottle. Shake well. Leave for 4 days to blend thoroughly.

Suggested uses:
• Massage into muscles after a warm bath or shower, and before strenuous or competitive sport.

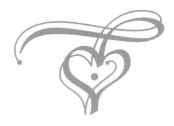

The After Sport Massage Oil is perfect to use after a heavy workout or game of sport

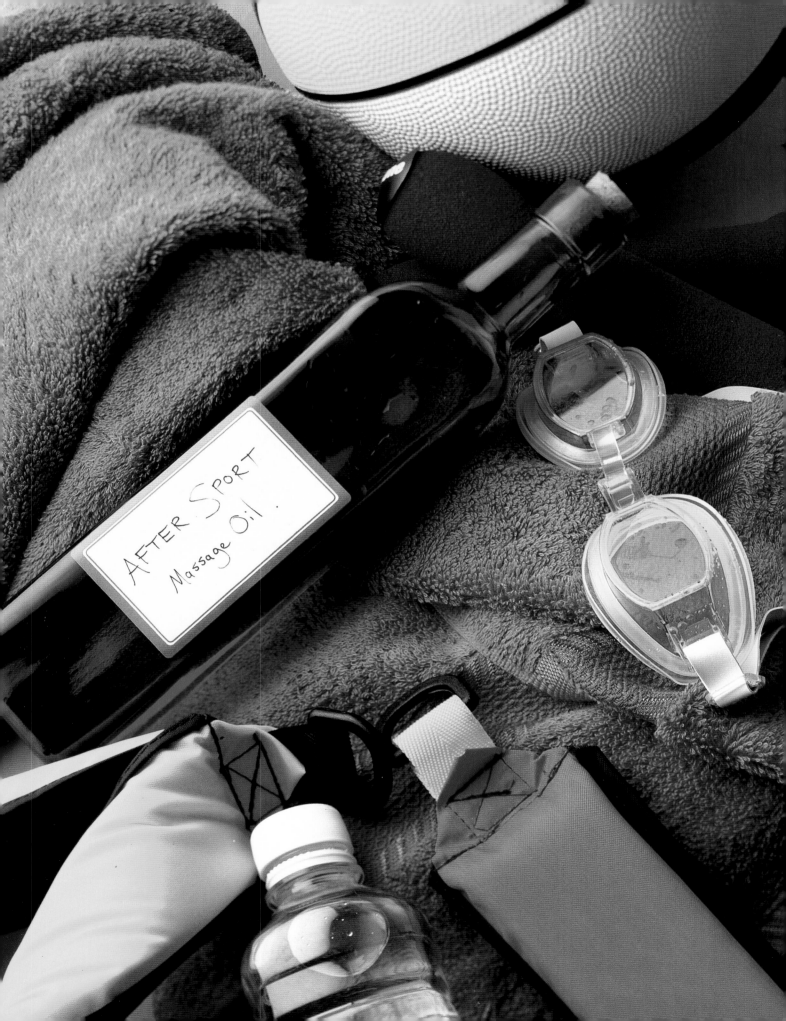

This massage oil will help to prevent or ease muscle soreness and also emotional soreness! When you arrive home, run a deep bath, pour a teaspoon of the oil blend into the bath and soak for half an hour. After drying off with a soft towel, massage some of the oil into your muscles.

> *100ml (3¹/₃fl oz) sweet almond oil, less 1 teaspoon*
> *20 drops rosemary oil*
> *20 drops lemon oil*
> *20 drops clary sage oil*
> *10 drops orange oil*

Mix all in a 100ml (3¹/₃fl oz) bottle. Shake well. Leave for 4 days to blend thoroughly.

Suggested uses:
- Use to massage muscles while in the bath or shower.
- Repeat the muscle massage after the bath or shower.

Travel and Holiday Stress

Your planned-for holiday, for which you have saved so diligently, can often turn into a very stressful experience. Here are a few precautions you may take to avoid this happening to you.

- A small, strong box containing a few essential oils is a must as part of your hand luggage. The oils will help you to avoid or treat many of the physical, mental and emotional problems.
- Plan well ahead. Try to avoid last minute panic situations. The night before you set off on your trip, make sure that the whole family sleep well by using one of the relaxing bath, massage or air spray blends found in this book.

Peppermint Tea

Travel sickness is both unpleasant and stressful. It can often be completely avoided by using this remedy.

1 teaspoon honey
1 drop peppermint oil
1 cup warm water

Mix the honey and peppermint oil and add to the warm water slowly, mixing constantly.

Suggested uses:
- Sip a cup of peppermint tea half an hour before leaving home.
- A bottle of this mixture can be taken with you in the car, boat or plane in case it is needed. Sip it: do not gulp. Do not drink more than 2 cups in 24 hours. Halve or quarter this amount for children, depending on age.

Aeroplane Travel

When you are flying to reach your holiday destination, there are a few simple rules to follow in order to arrive feeling as bright as possible and, hopefully, to avoid jet-lag.

- Drink plenty of water and fruit juice on the plane and try to avoid the temptation of the alcohol trolley, whether it is free or not!. If you feel nauseous, sip a little Peppermint Tea (above).
- Do not eat unless you are really hungry.
- Wear loose shoes or, even better, sandals as your feet will swell on a long journey. Spray or sponge your ankles and feet with water containing a few drops of lavender oil.

- Walk a lot. I resist the temptation to ask for a window seat as I try to walk at least every half hour and I do not want to irritate other passengers.
- Sprinkle a tissue with a few drops of eucalyptus oil. Breathe the scent deeply if you experience pain as the plane is descending. (This should not really happen if the crew are on their toes, as it means that they are not decompressing the cabin adequately.)
- Use the Fear of Flying? No Way! recipe below if you are really nervous.

Fear of Flying? No Way!

Many people are nervous of flying, even though statistically it is one the safest forms of transport. I suppose the fear comes from losing touch with the ground. If this fear is ruining your pre-holiday excitement, use the following essential oil blend for a week before you leave.

1 teaspoon bergamot oil
20 drops chamomile oil
2 teaspoons lavender oil
1 teaspoon geranium oil
80 drops sandalwood oil

Mix all the oils in a 25ml (approx. 1fl oz) bottle. Shake well. Leave for 4 days to blend thoroughly.

Suggested uses:
- In massage and bath oils.
- In an air spray and oil burner.
- As a toilet water splash.
- As a pulse point oil.
- Sprinkle 1 to 2 drops of this blend on a tissue or handkerchief, and inhale as needed.

Peppermint tea is a soothing
drink for travel sickness

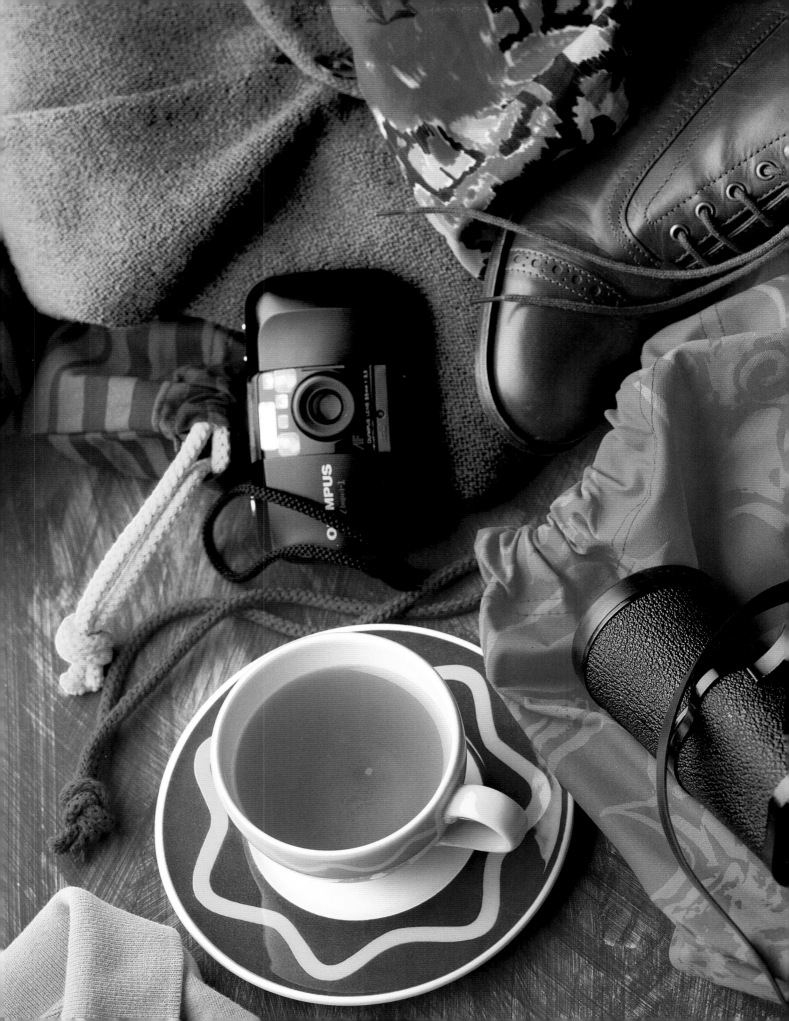

On Arrival

When you arrive at your hotel or holiday home, try to have a bath into which you have sprinkled 3 drops of lavender oil, 3 drops of geranium oil and 4 drops of grapefruit oil. If you cannot have a bath, sprinkle one drop of each oil onto a hot, wet flannel face cloth and use it in the shower.

It does not matter what time you arrive at your destination, try to stay awake until it is bedtime there. Sprinkle 1 drop of chamomile oil and 1 drop of lavender oil on a tissue and slip it inside the pillowcase to ensure a good sleep. This method will also soothe over-excited and fractious children.

Car Travel

If you are travelling with children, the biggest problem will be boredom. I used to say to my children: 'The last one to ask 'Are we nearly there?' gets a present!"

Stop every half an hour or so at parks, recreation areas and other suitable places. The time lost will be amply repaid in what will be a much happier journey.

Make up a little flask or bottle of Peppermint Tea in case of car sickness or nausea, and read the section 'On the Way to Work and School' for more suggestions on stress-free car travel.

Pre-operative Stress

There is bound to be a degree of nervousness and anxiety experienced before undergoing an operation. By using the following recipe, and the meditation technique described at the end of this chapter, you will be able to remain far more positive.

The Comforter

4 drops lavender oil
4 drops clary sage oil
2 drops ylang-ylang oil
2 drops chamomile oil

Mix all the oils in a 50ml (1²⁄₃fl oz) bottle. Shake well. Leave for 4 days to blend thoroughly.

Suggested uses:
- Make a 50ml (1²⁄₃fl oz) bottle of massage oil and toilet water using the above blend as the essential oils in each bottle.
- Use this oil blend on your pulse points, arms and legs.
- Sprinkle the toilet water on a wet flannel face cloth and wipe it gently over the body, face and neck after a shower or bath.
- Use the toilet water in a little atomiser to spray the face, neck and arms (avoid getting it in the eyes).

Post-operative Stress

Well, it is all over and you are on the road to recovery. Still, you may be feeling a little sore and tired, which can lead to depression and low spirits. This cheerful but gentle blend, will help.

4 drops lavender oil
4 drops grapefruit oil
2 drops mandarin oil
2 drops peppermint oil

Mix all the oils in a 50ml (1²⁄₃fl oz) bottle. Shake well. Leave for 4 days to blend thoroughly.

Suggested uses:
- See Pre-operative Stress.

Christmas!

There is a list of stressful situations which is used by psychologists and insurance companies, and it lists Christmas as a highly stressful occasion! Use the following essential oil blend to create calm amid chaos, and to fill the home or office with the warmly inviting, friendly and evocative scent of Christmas trees, pine cones and citrus groves.

Christmas Cheer

4 drops mandarin oil
4 drops orange oil
2 drops cedarwood oil
2 drops cypress oil

Mix all the oils in a 10ml (¹⁄₃fl oz) bottle. Shake well. Leave for 4 days to blend thoroughly.

Suggested uses:
- In air sprays or in oil burners.
- Pile a basket full of pine cones and sprinkle them with the oil blend. It will soak into the cones and make the room smell delicious, especially if they are placed in the hearth or in a sunny window where the heat will cause the oils to evaporate. Refresh the cones with more of the oil blend as needed.
- Sprinkle 1 drop only on each person's placemat before sitting down to eat. The heat from the plates will release the perfume.
- Sprinkle a few drops of the oil blend on the wrapping paper you are going to use, a week or so before Christmas. You will become calm and feel less stressed as you wrap the gifts, and the recipients will feel equally wonderful as they unwrap them.

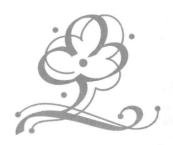

Christmas is a time of great stress for many, the perfect gift is an essential oil blend

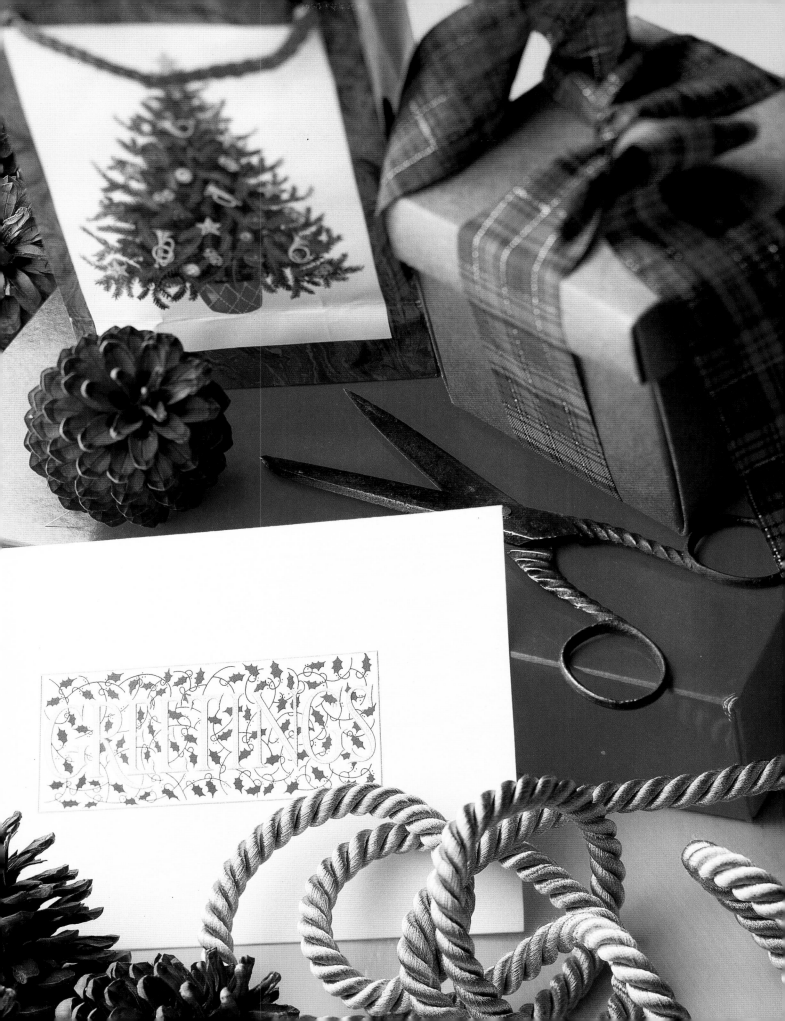

Premenstrual Syndrome (PMS)

So many women suffer from this distressing hormonal problem, and some are really incapacitated to different degrees. Essential oils are only part of a total strategy for this condition, but you may be agreeably surprised by the benefits you will receive from using a combination of the oils and other stress management techniques outlined in this book.

The PMS Chaser

2 teaspoons bergamot oil
½ teaspoon chamomile oil
½ teaspoon clary sage oil
1½ teaspoons geranium oil
½ teaspoon grapefruit oil

Suggested uses:
- Do not wait until you are feeling really bad. Use the oils every day.
- Include this blend in baths, after-shower treatments and massage oils.
- In air sprays and oil burners.
- As a pulse point oil and a toilet water splash.
- In the bedroom (see Bedrooms previously in this chapter).
- During meditation.

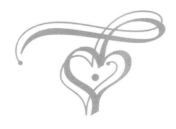

Menopausal Depression

Statistically, only about twenty-five per cent of women suffer unpleasant symptoms during menopause—but if you happen to be one of those twenty-five per cent, life can be pretty miserable. In this book, I am dealing only with the emotional and mental aspects of problems, and with menopausal symptoms there are obviously physical treatments which should also be pursued.

Beat the Menopausal Blues Blend

1 teaspoon clary sage oil
1 teaspoon geranium oil
1 teaspoon grapefruit oil
½ teaspoon peppermint oil
½ teaspoon lemon oil

Mix all the oils in a 25ml (approx. 1fl oz) bottle. Shake well. Leave for 4 days to blend thoroughly.

Suggested uses:
• See The PMS Chaser.
• Take a course of evening primrose oil capsules.

Pre-exam or Interview Stress

This stress can begin long before, and can become so severe that a successful outcome is threatened. Do not wait to take action.

No Brain-drain Blend

2 teaspoons bergamot oil
1 teaspoon grapefruit oil
½ teaspoon lemon oil
½ teaspoon lavender oil
1 teaspoon rosemary oil

Mix all the oils in a 25ml (approx. 1fl oz) bottle. Shake well. Leave for 4 days to blend thoroughly.

Suggested uses:
• See The PMS Chaser.

NOTE

The use of the Beat the Menopausal Blues Blend remedy, particularly when combined with meditation, has helped many people, myself included. It will help to ease the sweating and 'hot flushes', and the stress and embarrassment which accompany them.

Meditation

Cushion from Art Park, towel from Sheridan, flowers from Lisa Milasas

No book on stress and relaxation would be complete without a few words on meditation. Essential oils and meditation go hand in hand, and together can provide you with a sanctuary: a deeper, quieter space within where your problems become easier to solve or less important.

Put simply, meditation is the art of doing one thing at a time. You meditate if you are so immersed in what you are doing that time stands still and thought processes stop.

Meditation requires patience. It is a new skill which will happen slowly, in the same way as learning to play a musical instrument or a new language. Do not allow frustration to enter your meditation, or it will create the very situation you are seeking to resolve. Your mind has been allowed to do what it likes for your whole life so far, and at first it will resent any attempt to still the process.

There are many, many techniques for learning to meditate. There are plenty of good books to read on the subject and most towns offer meditation courses. The following method is a simple but effective one with which to begin and to enjoy this new experience. Please note that the key word is enjoy!

Meditation prevents you from
becoming overly stressed by
keeping a calm and peaceful mind

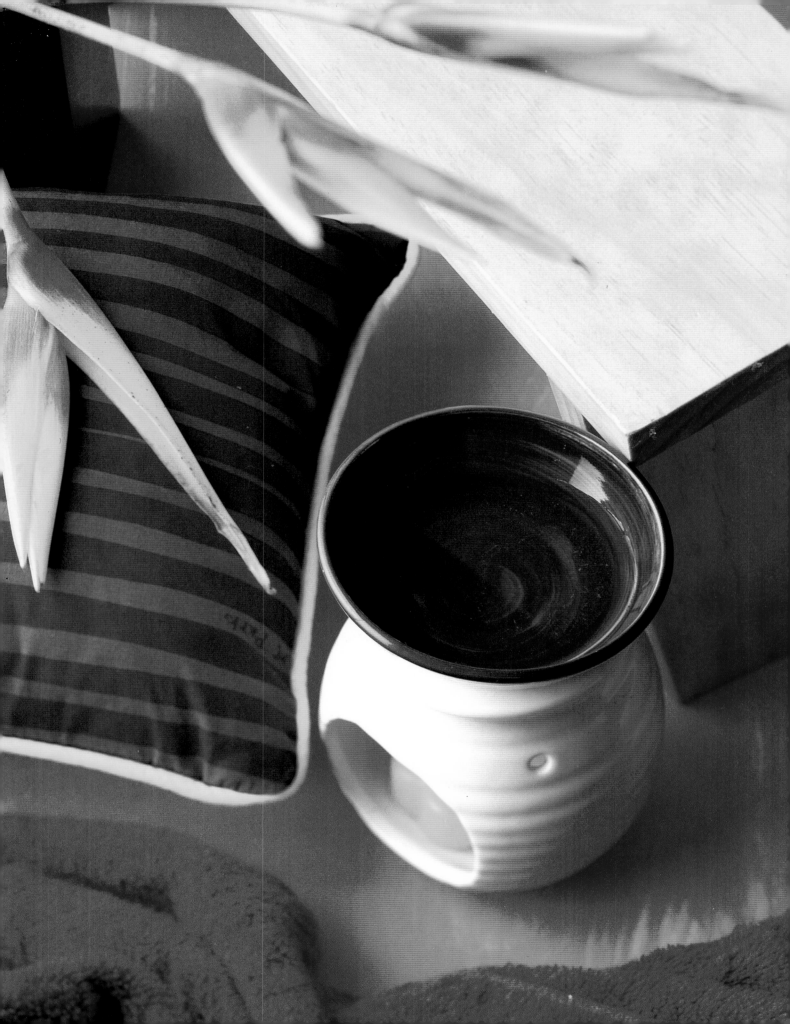

How to Meditate

The best times to meditate are early morning and in the evening, but any time is better than never.

Find a place where you can be alone. A corner of your bedroom, or the garden shed—even the car is quite a good place if your home is very noisy and full of people. Choose some quiet music, essential oils and comfortable clothes, and then you are ready to begin.

- Use the essential oil blend in an air spray, on pulse points, in an oil burner or sprinkled on cotton wool balls and placed nearby.
- Sit upright, but relaxed.
- Take a few deep, slow breaths, in through your nose and out through your mouth in a long, slow sigh. As you breathe out, let your muscles relax and imagine all muscular tension flowing out of your body with the breath.
- Let your shoulders drop, your jaw relax, the muscles around your eyes let go; let your stomach, thighs and buttocks become soft and slack. Do this for a few minutes…feeling a little better already? Now for the next step:
- Each time you breathe out, say 'one' in your mind and see the word 'one' on your 'mind-screen'.
- Breathe in gently—do not say anything.
- Breathe out, saying and seeing 'one'.

Continue for about 10 minutes to begin with. You will be able to increase the time as you become more at home with the process.

When thoughts intrude (which they will do continually!), do not become disheartened or feel you are a failure. Just push them gently but firmly to one side and return to 'one' and your breathing.

Meditation Blends

The 'One' Oil for Morning Meditation

2 teaspoons lavender oil
1 teaspoon bergamot oil
1 teaspoon sandalwood oil
½ teaspoon peppermint oil
½ teaspoon grapefruit oil

Mix all the oils in a 25ml (approx. 1fl oz) bottle. Shake well. Leave for 4 days to blend thoroughly.

Suggested uses:
• In a massage oil, and on pulse points.
• In an air spray or oil burner.

The 'One' Oil for Evening Meditation

1 teaspoon lavender oil
1 teaspoon geranium oil
1 teaspoon frankincense oil
1 teaspoon cedarwood oil
1 teaspoon bergamot oil

Mix all the oils in a 25ml (approx. 1fl oz) bottle. Shake well. Leave for 4 days to blend thoroughly.

Suggested uses:
• See The 'One' Oil for Morning Meditation.

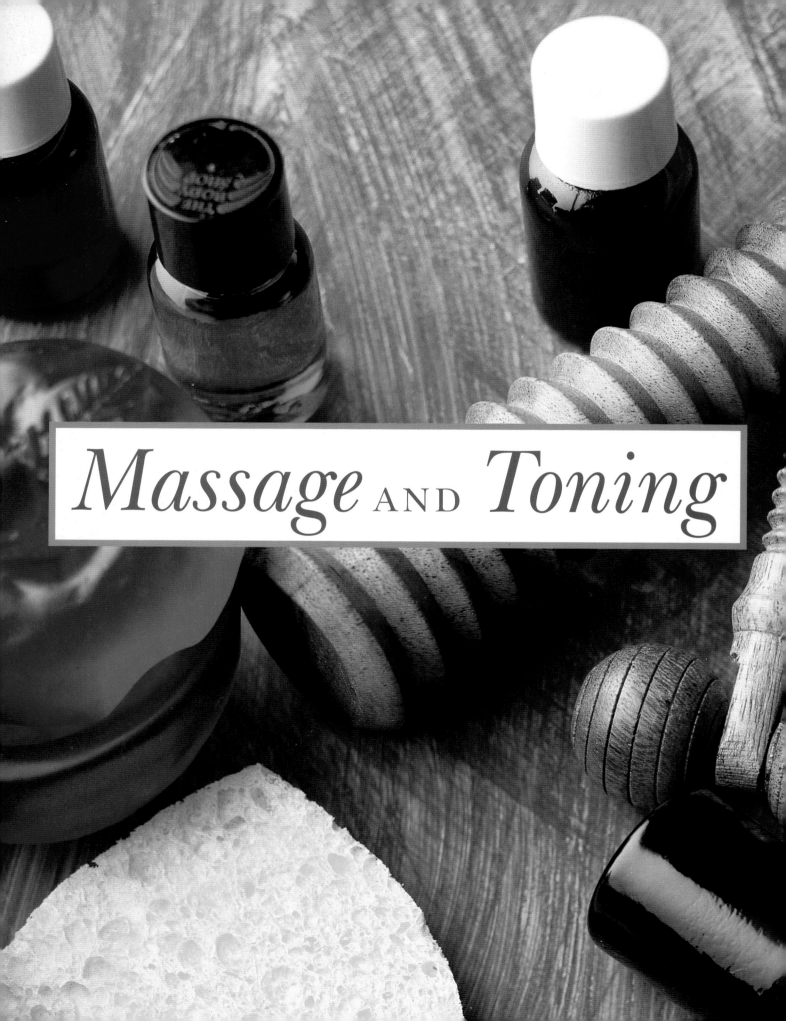

Massage AND Toning

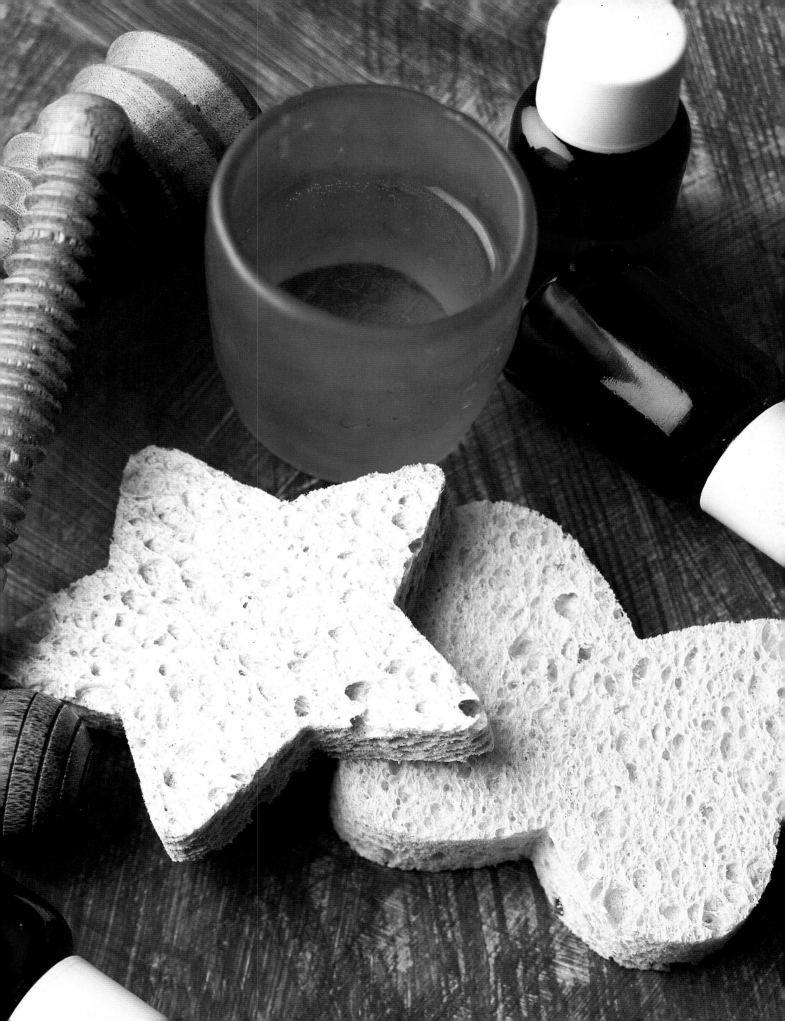

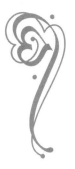

The History of Massage

For centuries, massage has been used as a therapy for healing and beautifying, as well as for improving body movement and general well being.

The Romans and Greeks used massage to treat their soldiers after battles and, during their training regimes, it was used for toning and stretching their bodies. Needless to say, the soldiers' battle-fatigued muscles benefited greatly from this ancient therapy.

The Chinese discovered the healing properties of massage very early on and they used it in conjunction with herbs, meditation, exercise and martial arts. The Chinese believed strongly in treating the whole person, not just an isolated symptom, and this belief has lasted and strengthened through the centuries until the present time.

Massage was used as a beautifying treatment by the ladies of ancient Greece. In ancient Rome, men and women alike enjoyed the public baths, followed by massages using sweet-scented oils.

Through past eras and the present, members of royalty have enjoyed receiving massages and several prominent physicians have employed massage as a complementary therapy to their medicine, with wonderful results. The herbalists of the past used herbal oils and balms in their treatments, a practice still used today.

The ever popular and relaxing Swedish massage was developed in the late 18th C. by Professor Peter Henry Ling, who first learnt of massage techniques during a trip to China and created this style of massage still used widely.

The Benefits of Massage

Massage has many benefits, not only to the skin, muscles and joints of the body, but also on a psychological level.

The many systems within the body respond to therapeutic massage. For instance, the circulatory system and the lymphatic system are both stimulated during a massage. This helps to improve blood flow through the body and also increases the elimination of built up toxins and waste materials.

The feeling of well being and relaxation you experience after a massage is due partly to the nervous system's many nerve endings being soothed and stimulated. The actual physical touch involved also has a soothing and comforting effect on the mind and body. Increasing the circulation of the blood promotes regeneration and repair of the skin, and also improves muscle tone and the general appearance of the skin.

Muscles respond rapidly to massage, and so it is excellent in sporting situations. Massage helps to stretch the muscles and so reduces aches and spasms; it also helps to speed the healing of strains and sprains.

Tension 'knots' are smoothed away, leaving a lighter feeling around the shoulder, upper back and neck area—an area particularly prone to aches and stiffness for many people. All types of work situations can bring stress to this area and cause spasms, which can lead to headaches and a feeling of tightness or pressure around the head.

Abdominal massage improves digestion and is beneficial for many digestive disorders, such as constipation and flatulence.

All in all, regular massage promotes a wonderful feeling of well being and lightness. The body and mind respond rapidly to this healing touch and many ailments are relieved or even disappear.

TIP

THE ART OF MASSAGE

To make sure that you, your family and friends enjoy the wonderful benefits of a massage with these aromatherapy recipes, I recommend that you learn the proper techniques. There are a number of excellent books which give step-by-step instructions and many places offer courses. I hope you enjoy learning about ways to use massage to enhance health and beauty.

Vase from Dinosaur Designs, flowers from Lisa Milasas

NOTE

Some essential oils are very toxic and should only be used internally on the advice of a qualified aromatherapist or naturopath. Many of the oils are unsuitable to use if certain conditions exist, such as epilepsy or pregnancy. Please note the cautions contained at the end of each relevant entry.

Essential Oils for Massage

There are few more pleasurable or healing experiences than receiving a massage, but this experience is immeasurably enhanced when essential oils are incorporated into the massage oil, cream or lotion.

The molecules of essential oils are small enough to pass through the skin. There, they dissolve readily into body fat, and are absorbed into the bloodstream and carried to all the systems of the body. The aroma of the oil is inhaled during a massage, affecting the limbic portion of the brain; they are also absorbed into the body through the lungs. Problems associated with the skin, such as poor circulation, muscular and joint problems, or problems to do with the digestive, genito-urinary, endocrine systems, immune and nervous systems may all be alleviated or healed through the use of essential oils.

The benefits of using the oils externally rather than internally are twofold. Firstly, the stomach is bypassed and the oils are not diluted or affected by gastric juices. Secondly, it is much safer to use the oils externally unless prescribed by an experienced person.

Most essential oils have healing properties, but some are more efficacious than others. The following list contains descriptions of 17 oils used in this chapter. The most useful massage oils are marked with an *. These marked oils are the best with which to start your 'aroma-massage collection'. They also have the advantage of being (with a couple of exceptions) the least expensive oils. The properties listed for each oil are only those applicable to healing.

If you can only afford a couple of oils to begin with, I would urge you to make lavender oil your first purchase, followed closely by chamomile oil and geranium oil. After you read through the recipes you will notice immediately how often these remarkable oils are used. Lavender, in particular, has the advantage of being gentle and safe enough to use for the whole family. I have not included the three oils which are among the most expensive, namely rose, neroli and jasmine. There are other less expensive oils which are very suitable for your purposes and which are far less costly.

*Essential oils are
the essences of plants*

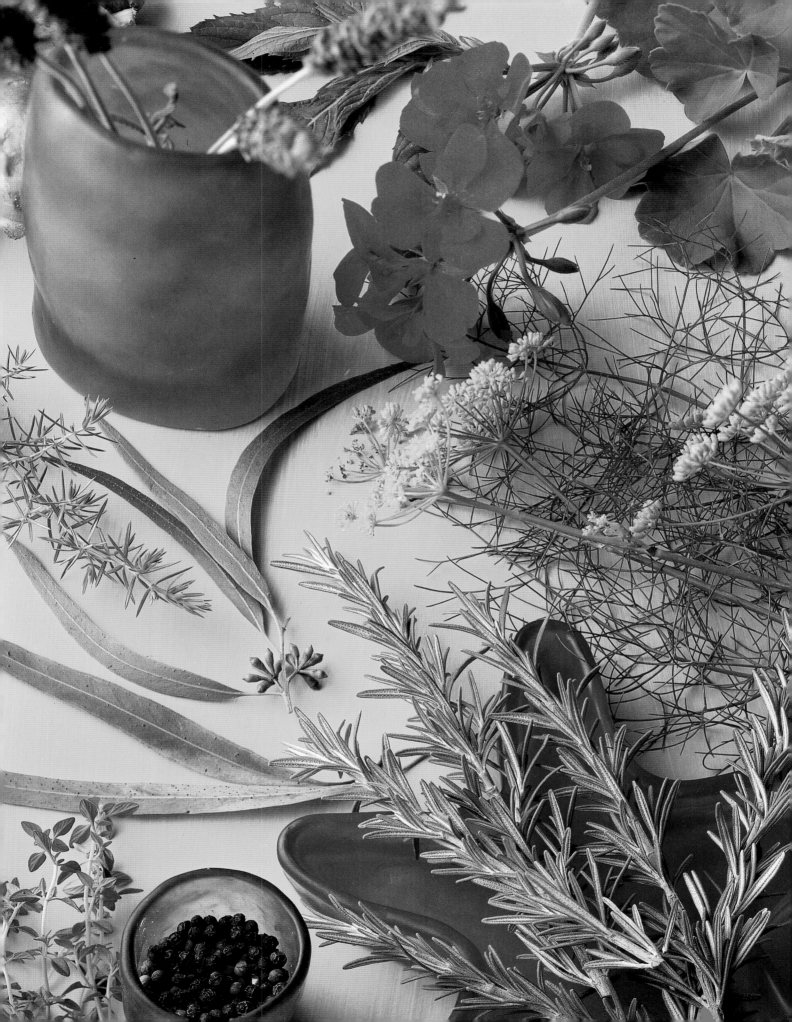

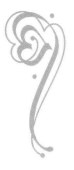

Black Pepper
Piper nigrum

MASSAGE APPLICATIONS: Arthritis and rheumatism, muscular aches and pains, sprains, and strains, muscular stiffness, neuralgia. Tones slack tissue and muscles, improves circulation. Pain-relieving and fever-reducing. May also be used for colic, constipation, diarrhoea, flatulence and nausea.

Cedarwood
Juniperus virginiana; Cedrus atlantica

MASSAGE APPLICATIONS: Antiseptic. Arthritis and rheumatism. Urinary tract problems. Bronchitis, coughs and catarrh. Nervous tension, mental exhaustion and stress-related problems.
CAUTION: Not to be used internally. Not to be used during pregnancy. An irritant to some sensitive skin types.

*Chamomile, German and Roman
Anthemis nobilis, Matricaria chamomilla

MASSAGE APPLICATIONS: Arthritis and rheumatism. Inflamed joints, flatulence, diarrhoea, headaches, insomnia, nervous tension, inflammation, sprains and strains. Menopausal problems. PMS. Ideal for babies and children.
CAUTION: A skin irritant to some people.

Cypress
Cupressus sempervirens

MASSAGE APPLICATIONS: Menopausal problems. Circulatory stimulant for cold hands and feet. Haemorrhoids, varicose veins. Coughs, laryngitis, colds. Muscle cramp, rheumatism. Oedema. Menopausal problems. Nervous tension. Muscle tone, back pain.

*Eucalyptus
Eucalyptus globulus and other species

MASSAGE APPLICATIONS: Muscular aches and pains, rheumatoid arthritis. Asthma, bronchitis, coughs, sinusitis, throat infections. Cystitis, leucorrhoea. Improves circulation and the immune system.

Fennel
Foeniculum vulgare

MASSAGE APPLICATIONS: Liver cleanser and digestive. Use for problems such as colic, constipation, indigestion, flatulence, nausea. Menopausal irregularities. Obesity (affects hormones), cellulite, fluid retention. Bruises, pyorrhoea. Asthma, bronchitis.
CAUTION: Phototoxic. Not to be used on skin before exposure to sunlight. Not to be used internally, in pregnancy or in epilepsy.

*Geranium
Pelargonium odoratissima and other species

MASSAGE APPLICATIONS: Acne, bruises, burns and scalds (minor), dermatitis, eczema, headlice, ringworm. Engorged breasts, menopausal problems, PMS. Poor circulation. Sore throat, tonsillitis. Wounds. Nervous tension, neuralgia.

Ginger
Zingiber officinale

MASSAGE APPLICATIONS: Arthritis and rheumatism, muscular aches and pains, poor circulation, sprains and strains. Catarrh, coughs, sore throat. Stomach cramp, nausea, travel sickness. Chills, colds, flu, fever. Nervous exhaustion.

Juniper
Juniperus communis

MASSAGE APPLICATIONS: Relieves urine retention. Removes toxins, gout, colds, flu, infectious diseases. Most period problems. Acne, dermatitis, eczema. Muscular pain. Anxiety, nervous tension.
CAUTION: Not to be used in pregnancy.

Jug, cups and jar from Dinosaur Designs, flowers from Lisa Milasas

*Lavender
Lavandula angustifolia
MASSAGE APPLICATIONS: Asthma, bronchitis, bruises, burns, sunburn and scalds (minor), catarrh, cystitis, depression, headaches, inflammations, insomnia, laryngitis, lumbago, muscular aches and pains, nausea, nervous tension, PMS, rheumatism.

Marjoram
Origanum marjorana
MASSAGE APPLICATIONS: Analgesic for arthritis, chilblains, lumbago, sprains, bruises, rheumatism, joint and muscle pain. Asthma, bronchitis, coughs, colds. Colic, indigestion, constipation. Headache, migraine, PMS.
CAUTION: Not to be used in pregnancy.

*Peppermint
Mentha piperita
MASSAGE APPLICATIONS: Asthma, bronchitis, colds, flu and fever. Colic, indigestion, nausea. Fainting, headache, mental fatigue, nervous stress, palpitations. Bad breath. Muscular pain, neuralgia.
CAUTION: Use in smaller quantities than other oils—1% is plenty. Never use during pregnancy.

Pine
Pinus sylvestris
MASSAGE APPLICATIONS: Arthritis and rheumatism, muscular aches and pains, poor circulation. Asthma, bronchitis, catarrh, coughs, sinusitis, sores, sore throat, colds and flu. Cystitis, urinary infections. Fatigue, nervous exhaustion.

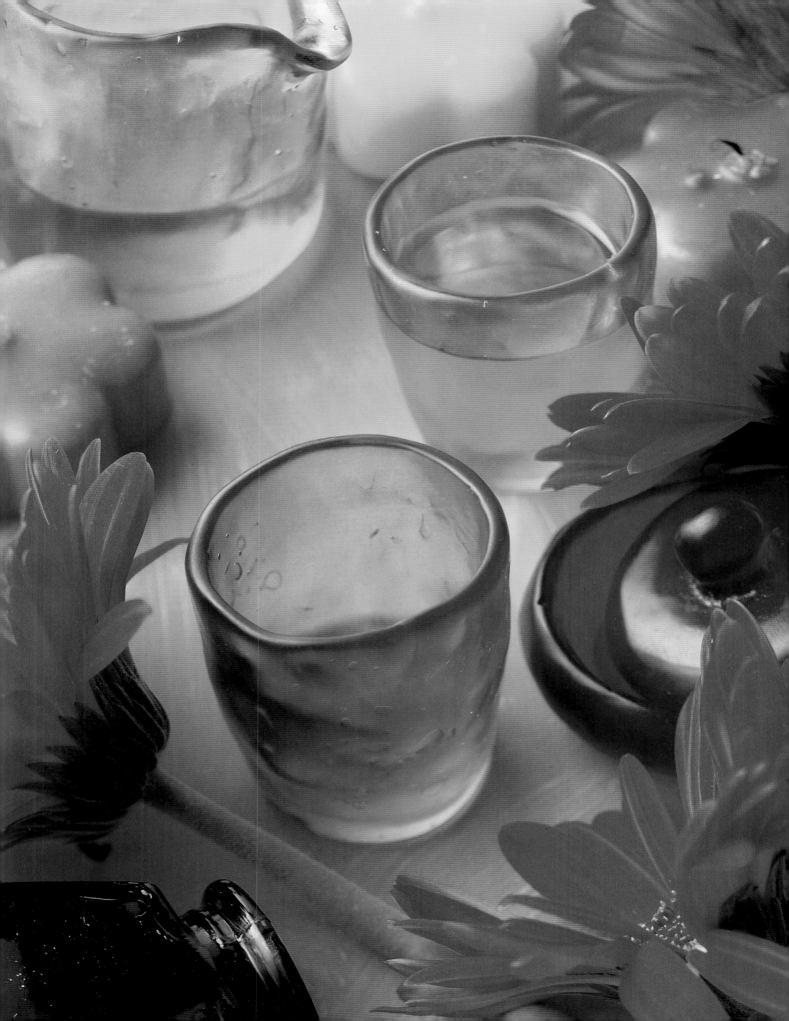

*Rosemary
Rosmarinus officinalis
MASSAGE APPLICATIONS: Arteriosclerosis. Asthma, bronchitis, colds, flu and fevers. Colitis, flatulence, fluid retention. Headaches, hypotension, infections. Liver problems. Nervous exhaustion, palpitations. Poor circulation, rheumatism, muscular pain, gout. Varicose veins. Whooping cough.
CAUTION: Not to be used in pregnancy or epilepsy.

*Spearmint
Mentha spicata
MASSAGE APPLICATIONS: The properties and uses of spearmint are similar to those of peppermint but are less powerful, making the oil more suitable for children.

Tea Tree
Melaleuca alternifolia and M. leucodendron
MASSAGE APPLICATIONS: A powerful antiseptic. Coughs, bronchitis, colds. Improves immune system response.

Thyme
Thymus vulgaris, T. citriodorus and chemotype linalol.
T. citriodorus and chemotype linalol are the safest to use for children as they are far less toxic than T. vulgaris.
MASSAGE APPLICATIONS: Arthritis and rheumatism. Asthma, bronchitis, catarrh, chills, colds and fevers, coughs, croup. Cystitis. Headaches. Infectious diseases. Insomnia, nervous debility, stress reliever. Improves immune system response.
CAUTION: A very powerful oil. Use only $\frac{1}{2}$–1%. Never use neat. Never use during pregnancy.

Special Recipes and Blends

Basic Massage Cream

This recipe is for a simple but very effective massage cream. The cream should not be refrigerated. Its thickness may be adjusted to your own preference, by using more or less oil.

30ml (1fl oz) olive or canola oil
125g (4oz) copha (hydrogenated coconut cooking fat)
5 drops simple tincture of benzoin
60 drops essential oil, chosen from an appropriate recipe

Melt the oil and copha together over a gentle heat. Remove from heat and allow to cool slightly. Beat in the mixed tincture and essential oil. Continue beating until cold. Pot in a clean glass jar.

Basic Massage Oil

The essential oils may be chosen according to the complaint being most frequently treated—see the following list for suggestions.

60ml (2fl oz) grapeseed or canola oil
1 teaspoon olive oil
3 teaspoons sweet almond oil
2 teaspoons avocado oil
1 teaspoon wheat germ oil (helps to prevent rancidity)
40 drops essential oil

Mix all the oils in a 100ml ($3\frac{1}{3}$fl oz) bottle. Add your choice of one of the following essential oil blends, and shake very well to mix. Leave overnight before use, shaking a few times more to blend thoroughly.

Aches and Pains, general

10 drops juniper oil
10 drops rosemary oil
10 drops lavender oil
5 drops black pepper oil
5 drops ginger oil

Mix essential oils together and add to 100ml ($3\frac{1}{3}$fl oz) of Basic Massage Oil. Shake well.

Arthritis and Rheumatism

10 drops chamomile oil
10 drops geranium oil
10 drops rosemary oil
5 drops black pepper oil
5 drops thyme oil

Mix oils, add to 100ml ($3^{1}/_{3}$fl oz) of Basic Massage Oil. Shake well.

Anti-cellulite

15 drops fennel oil
10 drops grapefruit oil
5 drops geranium oil
10 drops juniper oil

Mix oils, add to 100ml ($3^{1}/_{3}$fl oz) of Basic Massage Oil. Shake well.

Bruising

30 drops lavender oil
10 drops geranium oil

Mix oils, add to 100ml ($3^{1}/_{3}$fl oz) of Basic Massage Oil. Shake well.

Headaches

20 drops lavender oil
10 drops chamomile oil
10 drops rosemary oil
5 drops peppermint oil

Mix oils, add to 100ml ($3^{1}/_{3}$fl oz) of Basic Massage Oil. Shake well.

Immune System Booster

30 drops eucalyptus oil
5 drops thyme oil
5 drops tea tree oil

Mix oils, add to 100ml ($3^{1}/_{3}$fl oz) of Basic Massage Oil. Shake well.

Cup from Dinosaur Designs, flower from Lisa Milasas

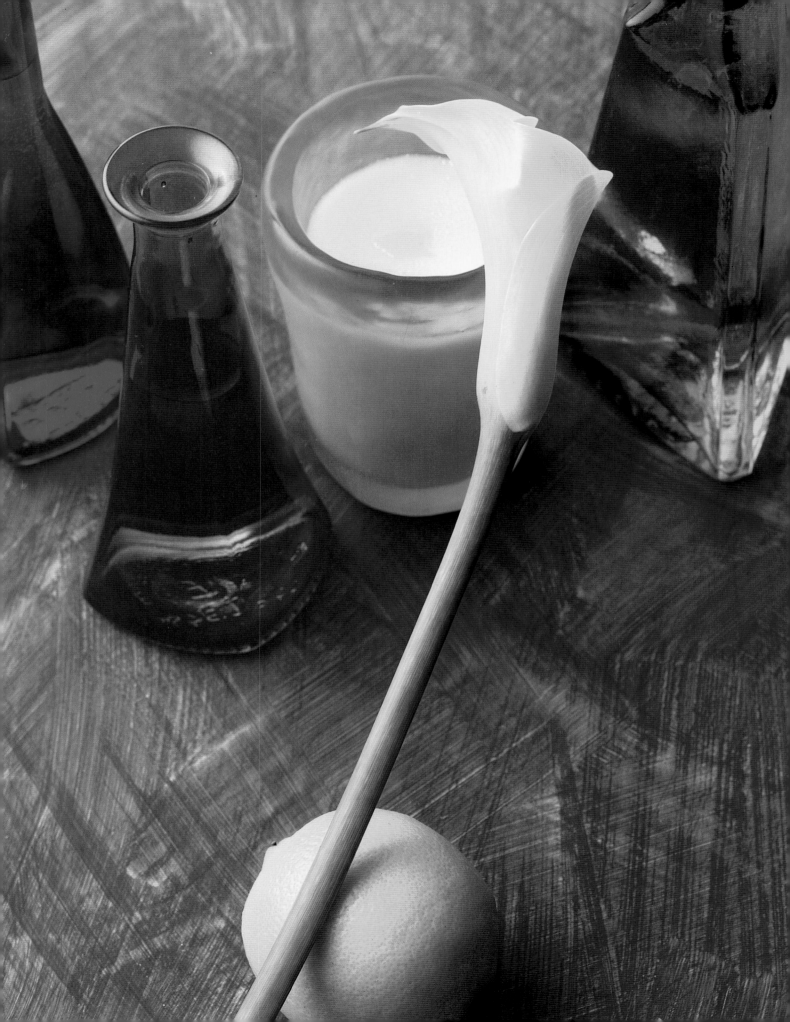

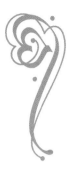

Menopausal Problems

20 drops geranium oil
15 drops cypress oil
5 drops fennel oil

Mix oils, add to 100ml (3¹⁄₃fl oz) of Basic Massage Oil. Shake well.

PMS (Pre-menstrual syndrome)

20 drops chamomile oil
10 drops geranium oil
10 drops lavender oil
5 drops marjoram oil

Mix oils, add to 100ml (3¹⁄₃fl oz) of Basic Massage Oil. Shake well.

Pregnancy

10 drops mandarin oil
10 drops lavender oil
5 drops chamomile oil

Mix oils, add to 100ml (3¹⁄₃fl oz) of Basic Massage Oil. Shake well.

Insomnia

20 drops chamomile oil
10 drops lavender oil
5 drops marjoram oil
5 drops sandalwood oil

Mix oils, add to 100ml (3¹⁄₃fl oz) of Basic Massage Oil. Shake well.

Mental Exhaustion

15 drops geranium oil
10 drops lavender oil
10 drops cedarwood oil
5 drops peppermint oil

Mix oils, add to 100ml (3¹⁄₃fl oz) of Basic Massage Oil. Shake well.

Nervous Tension

15 drops bergamot oil
10 drops lavender oil
5 drops cedarwood oil
5 drops sandalwood or frankincense oil
5 drops ylang-ylang oil

Mix oils, add to 100ml (3¹⁄₃fl oz) of Basic Massage Oil. Shake well.

Slack Tissue, to tone

10 drops grapefruit oil
10 drops marjoram oil
10 drops geranium oil
5 drops black pepper oil
5 drops juniper oil

Mix oils, add to 100ml (3¹⁄₃fl oz) of Basic Massage Oil. Shake well.

Babies, 2 days—2 years old

10 drops chamomile oil
3 drops lavender oil

Mix oils, add to 100ml (3¹⁄₃fl oz) of Basic Massage Oil. Shake well.

Children, 2 years—teenagers

10 drops chamomile oil
3 drops geranium oil
3 drops lavender

Mix oils, add to 100ml (3¹⁄₃fl oz) of Basic Massage Oil. Shake well.

Poor Circulation

15 drops rosemary oil
10 drops black pepper oil
5 drops ginger oil
5 drops lemon oil
5 drops eucalyptus oil

Mix oils, add to 100ml (3¹⁄₃fl oz) of Basic Massage Oil. Shake well.

Muscle Toner

10 drops rosemary oil
10 drops black pepper oil
10 drops cypress oil
10 drops juniper oil

Mix essential oils together and add to 100ml (3^1/3fl oz) of Basic Massage Oil. Shake well.

Back Pain

20 drops juniper oil
10 drops rosemary oil
10 drops cypress

Mix essential oils together and add to 100ml (3^1/3fl oz) of Basic Massage Oil. Shake well.

For Lovers

10 drops ylang-ylang oil
10 drops neroli or petitgrain oil
10 drops geranium oil
5 drops patchouli oil
3 drops bergamot oil
2 drops black pepper oil

Mix essential oils together and add to 100ml (3^1/3fl oz) of Basic Massage Oil. Shake well.

Coughs and Chest Problems

15 drops eucalyptus oil
15 drops cedarwood oil
5 drops pine oil
5 drops thyme oil

Mix essential oils together and add to 100ml (3^1/3fl oz) of Basic Massage Oil. Shake well.

To keep all your essential oils together, you can use a lovely timber box such as this

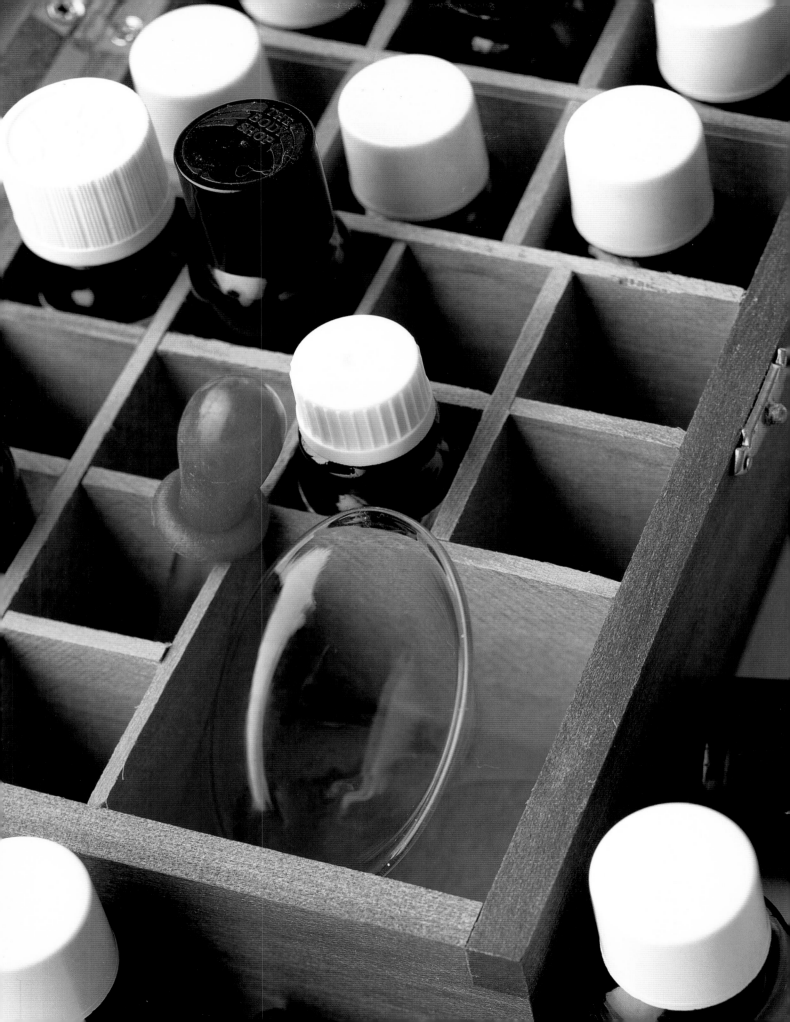

To centre yourself and become relaxed, light the oil diffuser and close the door while you are setting up the massage area. Then sit still for a few minutes and concentrate on breathing deeply and releasing the tension from your body with every out-breath. Put any problems you have on your mind aside to be dealt with afterwards. Stand and stretch, from toes to fingertips, and then you will feel peaceful and ready to give the massage. You will find this self-preparation helps immeasurably, not only for the recipient's enjoyment but also for your own.

Setting Up for Massage

A massage can be done on a massage table, a sturdy dining table or a spongy mat on the floor. It is easier to use a massage table although the dining table or floor are both more than adequate.

When choosing a massage table, make sure it is well-padded and set at a good height to work on; if it is too low, you, the masseur, could develop the backaches!

If you are using a dining table or the floor, it is important to lay down a thick padded surface, such as a covered foam mattress, a folded thick duvet or quilt, or several folded blankets. The person receiving the massage should feel as comfortable and as warm as possible. You will need several thick towels, one or two flat pillows and something soft for you to kneel on, if you are using the floor.

The atmosphere of the room is another point to consider. Soft lighting, soothing music and a blend of relaxing essential oils in an oil diffuser make a haven where relaxation is inevitable.

You will also find that the person being massaged will be much cooler than you. If the weather is cold, warm the room first and always ask if they are warm during the massage. Keep them covered at all times with the towels.

Giving a Massage

Once you are set up for the massage, you will need to consider several points for your own enjoyment and well being.

Your posture during the massage is of prime importance and you should assess it regularly. Keep a straight back and, if you need to bend lower, bend your knees and not your back. If you need to apply firm pressure, put your body weight behind your hands and the movement instead of relying on your arm and shoulder muscles to do all the work. Keep your shoulders relaxed and hold your stomach muscles in to help support your back.

It may seem a lot to remember at first but, once you have practised, it comes naturally. Any aches or stiffness in your own back are signals that your posture has not been correct.

It helps if you wear comfortable loose clothing and non-slip shoes if you are working on a bare floor. Your freedom of movement is important for your own comfort. Remove your jewellery and make sure your fingernails are short.

Try to avoid any interruptions. Alert other occupants of the house that you cannot be disturbed and, if necessary, switch on the telephone answering machine.

The next point to consider is your own state of mind. If you are tense, anxious or angry, you will not have a flow of positive energy between you and the recipient of the massage. He or she will sense these emotions and will also become tense. Do not underestimate this flow of energy: although it is subtle, it makes a huge difference between an ordinary massage and a wonderful one.

Cautions

In some instances it is wise not to give a massage, and some problem areas on the body should not be massaged. For instance:

- If the person has a fever or raised body temperature, it is best not to massage. However, you can massage their hands and feet, as this is quite comforting.
- Massage should be avoided when acute inflammatory conditions are present, such as arthritis, or wounds that are red and swollen, or any other condition where there is much swelling. Lightly massage the areas which are not affected, but not if they are below the swollen area; for instance, avoid giving a foot massage if the lower leg is badly swollen.
- In the presence of pus, such as ulcers on the body, boils and infected wounds, avoid massage altogether.
- Any abnormal skin conditions, such as burns, sores, scabies, ringworm or impetigo, should not be massaged. However, some oils are particularly useful for treating psoriasis and eczema.
- If the person has varicose veins, massage above the veins only. Gentle foot massage and light strokes are acceptable, but any firm massage below the veins causes more pressure and could cause complications or further inflammation of the veins.
- If a person has been bitten by a snake or spider, any form of massage will increase the flow of poison through the body. It is best to firmly bandage the area and keep it immobile until the person is able to reach a doctor.
- After recent bleeding in the body, such as the brain, stomach, lungs or bladder, it is best to avoid massage until the patient has the consent of their doctor.
- A person with thrombosis should not be massaged at all.
- Anyone with severe heart problems, such as left heart failure, should avoid any firm massage that increases circulation.
- Avoid massage if an organ or part of the body is inflamed, such as occurs in pancreatitis, meningitis, gastritis and appendicitis.
- Some essential oils are to be avoided in the case of epilepsy— these are mentioned in the Essential Oils for Massage section in this chapter.

NOTE

If the person has cancer, malignant tumours or tuberculosis, massage should be avoided. It is thought that the increased circulation of both blood and lymph that accompanies massage can increase the spread of cancerous metastasis through the body. Once again, a comforting foot, hand and head massage are usually safe, if these areas are not affected. Take care when massaging a woman within the first three months of pregnancy, depending on her history. Avoid any firm massage on the feet, as there are acupressure points on the feet which are used to induce labour. Use only very light massage on the abdomen and lower back.

Massage and Pregnancy

Sheet from Art Park

There are many essential oils that are not suitable for use during pregnancy. They are basil, cedarwood, clary sage, fennel, hyssop, juniper, marjoram, pennyroyal, peppermint, rosemary, thyme and citronella oils.

The first three months of pregnancy are when the most care must be taken with essential oils and massage. Never use the tapotement strokes—cupping, hacking and pounding—during the pregnancy. Do not use deep frictions or deep strokes of any kind around the lower back or abdomen during the early months. Use a smaller percentage of the safe essential oils in the massage oil blend.

To massage the back, it may be more comfortable for the person to lie on her side or to sit on a backward-facing chair, with a soft pillow between her abdomen and the back of the chair. When she is lying on her back at any stage during the massage, place a couple of pillows under her knees to provide support. Make sure she is comfortable before you begin. Follow the full body massage routine, omitting any frictions or deep strokes on the feet, abdomen and lower back. Omit any cupping, pounding and hacking. It is quite safe to use gentle frictions around the upper back, legs, arms and head.

Massage during the pregnancy helps to promote circulation, thus reducing the incidence of varicose veins, fluid retention and muscle cramps.

A gentle abdomen massage, omitting the deeper frictions and strokes, can be performed. This helps to ease constipation and indigestion, and it also reduces stretch marks by promoting the circulation of blood to the skin while the oils make the skin soft and supple.

By using gentle effleurage around the lower back area, the muscles will relax and this helps to relieve lower back pain. Further into the pregnancy, some firm effleurage and kneading of the lower back will be very beneficial. During the labour, back massage and firm foot massage will help ease discomfort and provides a source of relief.

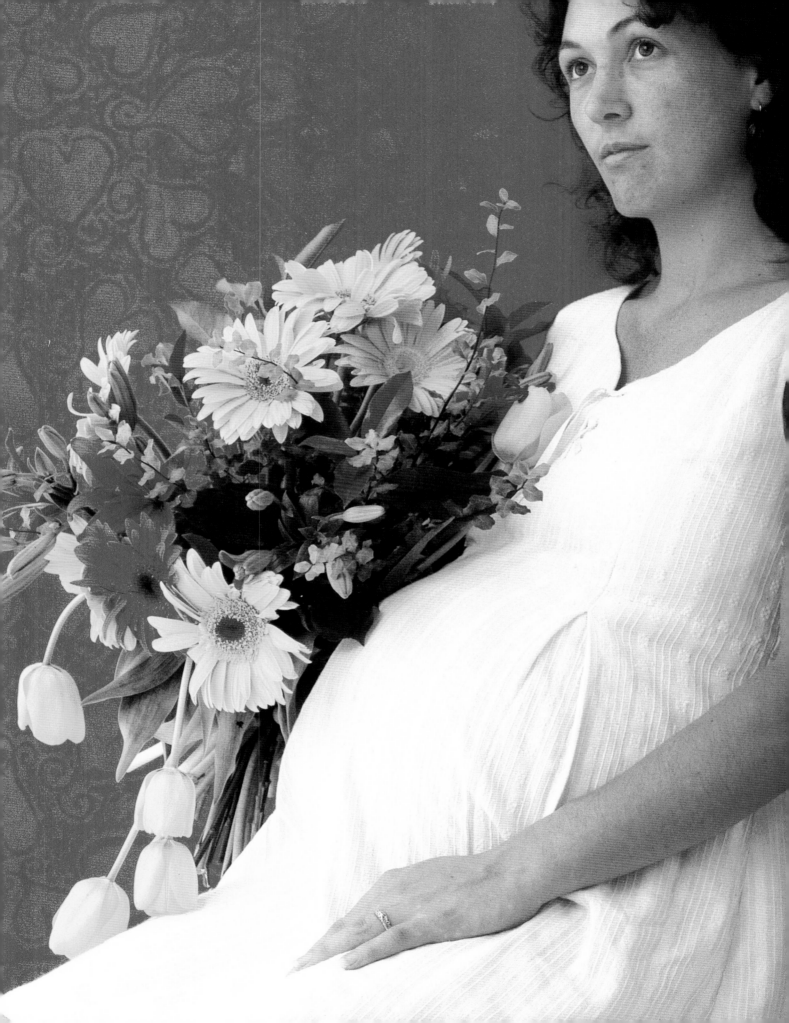

Babies and Children

Babies respond to touch naturally: they have not had time to develop any inhibitions or particular feelings against touching. Massaging will help to create a bond between the mother and father and the baby. If the baby is restless and colicky, massage will soothe and comfort, and so create a more peaceful baby.

Children can be massaged in the same manner as adults, except you use less pressure and not such deep strokes. Remember to be more gentle with the tapotement strokes of cupping, hacking and pounding, too.

Children also have muscle tension and aches from sports, bad posture or studying and doing homework for school.

Teach your children the correct posture for sitting at a desk and also while watching television. Bad posture overtaxes the muscles, creating spasms and aches.

Make sure if the child is doing exercise or sports that their instructor or coach teaches them to stretch their muscles before and after the activity to reduce muscle pain.

Towel from Sheridan, flowers from Lisa Milasas

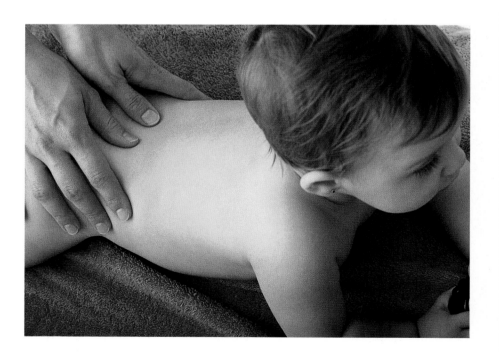

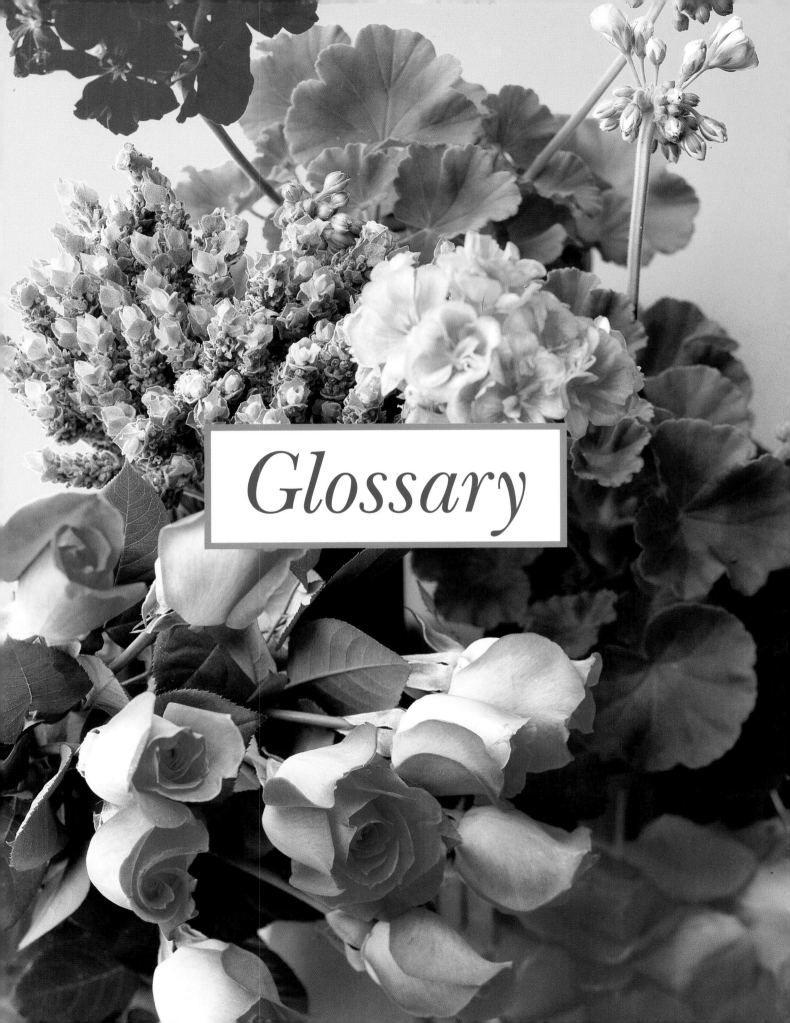

Glossary

Glossary of Terms

Allergen

Any substance which causes an allergic reaction. There is not a substance on earth which will not cause an allergic reaction on someone, but some substances are more likely than others to cause a problem. If you are allergy-prone or have sensitive skin, it would be wise to patch-test the essential oils before using them on your body.

To make a patch-test, add 1 drop of the oil you wish to test to 1 teaspoon of vegetable oil, and massage a little inside your elbow. Cover with a sticking plaster and leave for 24 hours. If there is no soreness, redness or irritation at the end of this time, you can safely go ahead and use the essential oil.

Almond oil, sweet

A fine, emollient, non-drying oil expressed from the kernel of the sweet almond (*Prunis communis dulcis*). An excellent oil to use in creams, lotions and massage oils formulated for dry, normal and combination skins.

Analgesic

A substance which is applied to lessen pain by exerting a nerve-numbing effect.

Antifungal

A substance which inhibits the growth of fungi. Fennel, myrrh, tea tree and thyme are antifungal.

Anti-inflammatory

A substance that reduces inflammation in the body or on the skin.

Antioxidant

A substance that retards deterioration by the process of oxidation, this can be of foods, skin products and within the body cells.

Antiseptic

A substance which inhibits the growth of bacteria on living tissue and prevents sepsis. tea tree and thyme oil are both powerful antiseptics.

Aromatherapist

A person skilled in the use of essential oils in the treatment of all types of ailments. They use the oils in massage, oil diffusers, compresses, etc. It involves intensive training to become a qualified aromatherapist.

Arteriosclerosis

A pathological condition of the circulatory system characterised by thickening and loss of elascticity of the arterial walls. The common name for this condition is hardening of the arteries.

Avocado oil

A beautiful thick, green oil. The oil contains the vitamins A, D, E and K, is rich, nourishing and invaluable in moisture creams and lotions, particularly for sensitive and sunburnt skins. the vitamin E content helps to preserve other oils in blends. Because of its thick consistency, it's best to use no more than 5–10% in massage and face oils.

Beeswax

A wax, secreted by bees, which forms the cell walls of the honeycomb. Beeswax is an ideal wax to use in ointments and creams. When combined with borax it makes an emulsifying wax.

It's possible to buy bleached white beeswax from pharmacies in pieces or in small buttons. I understand that it becomes hypoallergenic when treated in this way. It is however, very expensive and I like to use the natural untreated wax. Beeswax is a mild allergen.

Benzoin (Styrax benzoin)

Resin which is collected from incisions made in the bark of the tree and allowed to harden. The hard lumps of resin are then collected and used in many ways. They may be powdered in a pestle and mortar and used as a fixative in potpourri (add 10–30% by weight; that is, 10–30g ($^1/_3$–1oz) benzoin to 100g ($3^1/_3$oz) dried plant material); add to soap for the antiseptic, antibacterial and antifungal properties; made into a tincture and used as a preservative in creams, ointments and lotions. The tincture can be used as a topical application for eczema, blackheads, boils, pimples and itching.

Note: If you buy the tincture from a pharmacy be sure that you buy only Simple Tincture of Benzoin. Compound tincture of benzoin (also known as Friar's Balsam) has other additives which may be harmful if used incorrectly.

Canola oil

Canola seed is modified rape seed. Rape seed oil has been under a cloud due to the presence of eructic acid which, when eaten in large quantities showed a fat accumulation in the heart muscle of animals. Canola was bred to be genetically low in eructic acid. This process was carried out in Canada hence the first three letters of the name.

Canola is a non-drying oil which is excellent in massage oils and in creams and lotions for dry and normal skins. It is also good for cooking as it is light and has little flavour of its own. If you like the taste of butter but don't want to eat so much saturated fat you could beat some canola oil into softened butter. This gives a spreadable consistency, less saturated fat and the benefits of monounsaturated fat. Unfortunately it still has the same number of kilojoules (calories)!

Carbuncle

This is a painful skin eruption, similar a boil but quite large, with several openings; caused by a staphylococcal infection.

Catarrh

Involves an inflammation of a mucous membrane with an increased production of mucus. Especially affects the nose and throat in the common cold virus.

Cellulite

Is a build up of subcutaneous fat that creates a dimpled effect under the skin. Usually found on the buttocks, thighs and hips. The best way to deal with cellulite is to eat a wholesome natural diet with lots of fresh fruit and vegetables, drink 6–8 glasses of purified water a day, maintain a healthy weight, exercise often and regularly have massage (or use self-massage techniques) using essential oils to help break down and remove cellulite (see recipe in the Massage and Toning chapter).

Chilblains

Some people are susceptible to chilblains on the toes, fingers and ears. They are usually caused by exposure to cold and moisture and result in inflammation of the skin. They are quite painful and should not be exposed to high heat as this causes further irritation. Keeping the fingers and toes warm with wool gloves and socks helps to reduce the chilblains.

Colic

This is a condition characterised by acute spasmodic abdominal pain. It is usually caused by inflammation and distention of the gastrointestinal tract. A baby with this condition can cry for the first 3 months of life and will eventually grow out of it.

Compress

A method of applying heat, cold, stimulation, moisture or the healing properties of various agents to areas of the body. See the Health and Healing chapter for more information.

Conjunctivitis

An inflammation of the conjunctiva of the eye. The symptoms can include stinging, pus, a red appearance of the eye and a watery discharge.

Copha

A white hydrogenated coconut oil product. The hydrogenation causes the oil to become solid. Do not substitute with margarine.

Cornflour

Cornflour can be made from maize or wheat. It acts as a thickening agent.

Digestive

An agent which aids digestion. An example is peppermint oil.

Disinfectant

A substance which destroys bacteria and so helps to prevent disease.

Effleurage

A firm and flowing massage technique used to calm the recipient, apply oil and warm the muscles ready for more intense massage strokes.

Essential oil

The concentrated essence of a plant usually obtained as an oil by steam distillation.

Expectorant

A substance that help to expel sputum from the respiratory tract. Useful for colds, flu, bronchitis etc.

Fistula

This is an abnormal opening between one hollow organ of the body and another, or between a hollow organ and the skin caused by ulceration or congenital abnormalities.

Frictions

A firm massage stroke which helps to relieve muscle spasm.

Fomentation

The use of hot wet cloths to ease pain and reduce inflammation.

Glycerine

Glycerine is a natural substance present in animal and vegetable fats. It is usually obtained as a by-product of soap making. It is syrupy in consistency, colourless, odourless, sticky and sweet. If used in small proportions in lotions, creams and toners it acts as an antibacterial, softener, lubricant and humectant (holding moisture to the skin). If more than twenty per cent is used in any recipe it will have the opposite effect and draw water from the skin. Adding a little glycerine to colognes gives a soft feeling to an after-shower splash.

Glycerine acts as a preservative but in order to be effective it needs to be present as twenty per cent of the total content, which would be far too much for most recipes; however, even a small amount will help preserve to some degree, particularly if combined with four per cent tincture of benzoin.

Grapeseed oil

As the name suggests, this oil is pressed from grape seeds. It's a fine, semi-drying, polyunsaturated oil which makes it suitable for most skins except the very oily. It is a very good basic carrier oil as it is light, clear and has no smell. Add five to ten per cent wheat germ oil to help prevent rancidity.

Hydrogenation

A process using hydrogen by which liquid oils are converted into solid fats such as margarine. Hydrogenation produces abnormal EFA (essential fatty acids) — these are mirror images of normal EFA. The body accepts these abnormal EFA and attempts to use them but by the time it finds that the atoms of the molecules are arranged in the wrong 'shape', the process has gone too far to abandon them and begin again with normal EFA; the normal EFA are blocked out. The end result of this process is that by the use of hydrogenated products we are depriving the body of EFA. According to the British medical journal *Lancet*, 'The hydrogenation plants of our modern food industry may turn out to have contributed to the causation of major disease'.

Hyper-pigmentation

Excessive skin pigmentation caused by over-exposure to sun or use of plants or oils which cause photo-sensitivity. Bergamot oil is one.

Impetigo

This contagious bacterial skin disease is represented by the formation of pus blisters that develop into crusty scabs with a yellow colour.

Insomnia

There are many causes of insomnia—stress, overeating, alcohol and more. Several of the essential oils will help to promote sleep and relaxation. Lavender, chamomile and sandalwood are a few of these oils and can be used in a massage oil or in an oil diffuser.

Lanolin, anhydrous

Also known as 'wool fat'. This is a sticky yellow grease obtained by boiling the shorn wool of sheep. Lanolin is often sold as hydrous lanolin which means that water has been beaten into the lanolin to make it more spreadable. The Healing Ointment recipe contains anhydrous (no water added) lanolin.

I stopped using lanolin for some time because of the many chemicals which were poured on the sheep's back. The new methods of treating sheep have resulted in purer lanolin but there will still be a pesticide residue in the wool fat if the sheep have grazed on pasture which has been treated with organophosphates, as these are deposited in the fat of both animals and humans and are cumulative. Much work is apparently being done on producing biodegradable pesticides which wouldn't present the risks to health that the present ones pose (unless you happen to be a ladybird, frog, praying mantis etc!! I still can't come to terms with the use of pesticides and herbicides on such a widespread scale).

The Food and Drug Authority has stated that the acceptable levels of pesticides in lanolin should be no more than five parts per million and this standard is one which is being used in Australia. I now feel that lanolin is probably a safer choice healthwise than petroleum jelly but I would recommend that nursing mothers could try substituting cocoa butter and coconut oil in nipple creams instead of lanolin. Allergen.

Leucorrhoea

A vaginal infection with the symptoms of a white to yellow discharge.

Naturopath

A person qualified in the treatment of other by employing natural methods including herbal medicine, nutrition, homeopathy, massage and lifestyle counselling.

Neuralgia

A severe pain caused by nerve damage or malfunctioning.

Oedema

The swelling of tissue that can be due to many causes.

Oils

See the individual oils.

Olfactory system

The system in the body responsible for the sense of smell.

Olive oil

A rich non-drying oil expressed from ripe olives. It is one of my favourites and I use cold-pressed Extra Virgin (how on earth can you have 'extra' virgin—you either are or you aren't!) which is from the first pressing and is very green and aromatic. Some people don't like the smell so maybe they could try one of the lighter olive oils from later pressings.

Olive oil is too rich for oily skins but is excellent for massage oils, creams, soaps and lotions for dry and normal skins. A lovely oil to use on the skin of babies.

Palpitations

A condition where the heart feels as though it is 'racing'. It can be caused by a variety of factors.

Petrissage

A massage stroke used to knead a muscle to help relieve spasm and tension. It is done rythmically and firmly.

Photo-sensitivity

See Hyper-pigmentation.

Poultice

A pulped, heated mass of herbs, vegetables or other agents usually enclosed in cloth and applied to the skin to relieve congestion or to draw pus or foreign bodies from a wound.

Pruritus

This condition is one of intense itching.

Pyorrhoea

This dental disease has symptoms of pus or discharge and loosening of the gums.

Rancidity

Many fats and oils can become rancid or 'go off'. The addition of an antioxidant such as vitamin E oil and also refrigerating the product can increase the shelf life.

Rose-water

A scented water made from rose petals or rose oil. Triple rose-water (which may be bought from pharmacies) is prepared by distillation of fresh blooms of *Rosa damascena*. To use, add one part rose-water to two parts purified water. The resulting rose-water can be used in cleansing creams, toners, moisture lotions and as a toilet water.

Scabies

A mite causes this very contagious skin infection. A person with scabies will experience intense itching, inflammation and small blisters

Spasm

Muscle spasms can occur due to overuse, stress and also from using a muscle not exercised very often.

Sprain

A sprain is a joint injury and is caused by twisting the joint and injuring the ligaments around that joint.

Strain

This is a muscle injury caused by over-exertion. The muscle can tear creating much pain and swelling.

Styptic

An agent which helps to control external bleeding. Witch hazel extract, cypress oil and lemon oil are styptic.

Talcum, unperfumed

A mixture of various chalks which are milled until very fine. It's most important to use only pharmaceutical standard, sterilised talcum—earthborne bacteria such as tetanus may be contained in unsterilised chalk. These bacteria could cause illness and in the case of small babies, death. Sterilise dubious talcum in a 150°C (300°F) oven for one hour, stirring often.

Tapotement

A massage stroke used to stimulate the body and will help to promote circulation of blood and lymph through the body.

Tincture

A method of preserving the properties of herbs by extraction into an alcoholic solution.

Vinegar

The word 'vinegar' is derived from the French vin aigre which means sour wine. Cider vinegar is made from apples, and wine vinegars from grapes; these are the two most suitable for cosmetic use. Malt and other vinegars are too harsh for use on skin.

Water

Water is a good medium for the growth of bacteria and, as water is used frequently in the treatments in this book, it is necessary to use purified or distilled water where specified to ensure that the remedy is as pure as possible.

Wheat germ oil

This is a richly nourishing fine, healing oil. The vitamin E content makes it useful for most skins, especially dry, prematurely aged skin or for skin troubles such as eczema or psoriasis. Good in 'anti-stretch mark' blends. Helps to preserve other oils. Ten per cent is a valuable addition to creams and lotions, massage oils and soaps.

Witch hazel (Hammamelis virginiana)

Distilled witch hazel extract. In this book you will find many remedies using witch hazel for its astringent and styptic properties. It helps to reduce skin inflammation, the pain of stings, bruises and swellings. Distilled witch hazel is readily available from pharmacies.

Wool fat

See Lanolin

Zinc oxide powder

A soft, heavy, white powder which when added to creams forms a soothing, mildly astringent protective barrier. Very suitable for application to babies' bottoms.

HINT

FURTHER READING

AROMATHERAPY,
Robert Tisserand
(Granada, 1977).

THE PRACTICE OF
AROMATHERAPY,
Jean Valnet, MD
(Healing Arts Press, 1980).

AROMATHERAPY,
Nerys Purchon
(Hodder Headline Australia
Pty Limited, 1994).

THE FRAGRANT PHARMACY,
Valerie Ann Worwood
(Bantam Books, 1991).

THE COMPLETE HOME
GUIDE TO AROMATHERAPY,
Erich Keller
(Munchen, 1991).

THE ENCYCLOPAEDIA
OF ESSENTIAL OILS,
Julia Lawless
(Element Books, 1992).

THE DIRECTORY
OF ESSENTIAL OILS,
Wanda Sellar
(C.W. Daniel Company
Ltd, 1992).

THE ENCYCLOPEDIA
OF AROMATHERAPY,
MASSAGE AND YOGA
Carole McGilvery,
Jimi Reed, Mira Mehta
(Acropolis Books, 1993).

MASSAGE
Denise Brown
(Headway. Hodder &
Stoughton, 1993).

AROMATHERAPY
FOR HEALING THE SPIRIT,
Gabriel Mojay
(Hodder &
Stoughton, 1996).

Index